Help! My Child's Anxiety is Giving Me Anxiety

Saskia Joss is a child and adolescent therapist specialising in anxiety and trauma at the Mill Hill Therapy Hub. Originally a primary school teacher at a range of London schools, she retrained as a therapist and has since worked across multiple state schools and in private practice, supporting children and families. Since Covid-19, Saskia has become a leading voice on childhood anxiety, helping families navigate the mental health challenges arising from lockdowns and isolation. An acclaimed international lecturer on anxiety, early years education, psychoeducation and parenting, she is also a regular guest on television and radio, advocating for children's mental health.

Help! My Child's Anxiety is Giving Me Anxiety

Saskia Joss

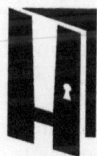

First published in 2025 by Headline Home
An imprint of Headline Publishing Group Limited

1

Cataloguing in Publication Data is available from the British Library

Hardback ISBN 978 1 0354 2410 8
ebook ISBN 978 1 0354 2412 2

Typeset in 14/18.5pt Dante MT Std by Jouve (UK), Milton Keynes

Printed and bound in Great Britain by Clays Ltd, Elcograf S.p.A.

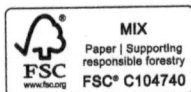

MIX
Paper | Supporting responsible forestry
FSC® C104740
FSC www.fsc.org

Headline's policy is to use papers that are natural, renewable and recyclable products and made from wood grown in well-managed forests and other controlled sources. The logging and manufacturing processes are expected to conform to the environmental regulations of the country of origin.

Headline Publishing Group Limited
An Hachette UK Company
Carmelite House
50 Victoria Embankment
London EC4Y 0DZ

The authorized representative in the EEA is Hachette Ireland,
8 Castlecourt Centre, Dublin 15, D15 XTP3, Ireland (email: info@hbgi.ie)

www.headline.co.uk
www.hachette.co.uk

To my wonderful children, Amiel and Cecily, I love you so much and will love you forever. I hope you can see how hard I am trying to make this world safe and magical for you.

To my re-Marc-able husband, thank you for making me feel safe and supported strongly enough to be brave.

To the parents who are trying to help their children unleash their potential, flourish and thrive, I salute you and stand with you always by your side.

Contents

Prologue

HI THERE,

My name is Saskia and 'You are welcome here!' Whether you have one child or ten, whether you parent alone or in a team, whether you're worried about your youngest, oldest or only child, you are welcome. You are now part of my team and it is a pleasure to have you.

All the parents I work with in my therapy practice are aiming to get through the long days of their little one's early childhood with as few broken nights and broken bones as possible. They are hoping to see their child hand in hand with other children, joining in and having fun.

It seems like a simple goal, but if you are reading this book, you will know it isn't always straightforward. On the days when your wailing two-year-old won't let go of your leg and trot happily into the Montessori nursery you had to put them down for at birth; when at 10 p.m. after a magical day at

Legoland your six-year-old tells you he is too scared of dying to sleep; or when your nine-year-old rings you, hyperventilating, pleading to be collected from the sleepover she's been begging to attend for weeks – on those days it is hard not to think that all your parenting choices have been deeply flawed. Welcome to a tidal wave of anxiety as you realise that, with the best will in the world, you don't know what to do next.

We've all been there!

Help! My Child's Anxiety is Giving Me Anxiety!

This is where I come in, holding this book, probably sipping a cup of tea with oat milk in it, giving you a reassuring smile. Rest assured I am armed with all you need to know to get through the most anxiety-making moments in parenting.

When I was a child and people asked me what I wanted to be when I grew up, after saying I fancied whizzing around on roller skates and appearing in *Starlight Express*, I'd say I wanted to be a well-wisher.

Yes, you read that correctly. I wanted to be a well-wisher, which I would explain involved shouting my congratulations at a happy wedding, bringing the ma'amoul to a sensational Eid celebration, attending a minimally visited funeral or clapping for someone after a great first day in a new job as an estate agent. It sounds like a service few would take up, but for me it was about the idea of supporting people with kindness and positivity; being a useful, visible face at a time when it's nice to be seen.

Let me just get it out of my system . . . I wish you well too! I guess that you have bought this book because you are feeling lost and overwhelmed by your anxiety or your child's or both. You are looking for something to bolster you and your family and help you enjoy and experience life as it is meant to be.

I am planning to do just that with my expertise, information and practical ideas, all grown and gleaned from my real years on the ground and in the trenches.

Here's how I got here:

After years of running summer camps, after-school clubs and babysitting (having given up on well-wishing as a career choice), no one was surprised when I qualified as a primary school teacher. I became a reception class teacher in a one-form entry school in north London. Nothing made me happier than staring down at thirty tiny smiley faces, singing songs, teaching reading and giving children the happiest, most fun start to learning they could have. When I had to say goodbye to my first class at the end of my Newly Qualified Teacher year, I cried for two days straight. I had loved it and loved them. It was such a privilege to get a year with these mini minds and teach them things I had learned at my creative school or from my own poetry-reading, story-performing mum.

The pain and pressure of making an impact in only one year and then handing my teeny colleagues on to a different teacher felt awful. What if the new teacher shouted at them and didn't let them go to the loo until break time, even though they were only just out of nappies? Even as I bonded with the next group, I knew that I couldn't be a teacher forever.

I decided to requalify to become a person-centred therapist for adults. I studied in the evening while working full time. Person-centred therapy, started by Carl Rogers, sets out from the premise that no one can know you as well as you do. It was a new dawn for therapy; the therapist was no longer the all-knowing tour guide of your soul, who was doing you a favour by taking all your cash, assessing you from on high and occasionally bestowing a crumb of judgement that would send you into a tailspin.

Person-centred therapy is more like hiring a friendly, chatty cabbie who is interested in getting to know you while you get to choose which route your subconscious will take. It's supportive, loving and positive, as well as being quicker and more goal-orientated than analysis. It helps people to see what a fair, equal relationship is like where you can feel valued and important without shame. Above all, it aims to help people feel more like themselves and feel proud: the goal is deep self-awareness but also happiness. I loved my course – I trained at the CPPD in Alexandra Palace, London and it was a revelation. As a small teaching group of sixteen, we learned all sorts of therapeutic theory, including Gestalt therapy, Maslow's hierarchy of needs and transactional analysis, as well as the principles of person-centred therapy.

As I finished the course, I also got a new job at the Orion Primary School, one of the biggest primary schools in London, run by the revolutionary head Christopher Flathers, a winner of the Pearson Headteacher of the Year award. Chris is an inspirational super head running a four-form primary school with a large unit attached for children on the autism spectrum. His mantra is that children have to be happy to learn and he sets about making a school that is so happy it gives Disneyland a run for its money.

The adults at the Orion are hired because they are talented but also because they are good, kind people who invest in the community and its success. It was glorious but inside I felt this amazing pressure to give these children all I could. I was doing everything I was told and using the special jargon Chris invented like a native. But I was sure however well I taught the phonics or loudly I clapped in Chris's jamboree-style assemblies that, as a teacher, I couldn't do enough to swing the balance back to a fair start for some of these children.

So, I changed my plan again. I began to retrain to become a therapist for children. I studied under world expert Margot Sunderland at the Institute for Arts in Therapy and Education and happily surrendered my weekends for a year as I was learning things that changed my life, my teaching and eventually my parenting too!

It was like swimming in magic. The institute had a careful focus on neuroscience as Margot had been trained by the late visionary Jaak Panksepp, the father of 'affective neuroscience', which explores the science behind emotions in the brain. As Margot was a big name in child therapy, she brought the biggest names to us. There were personal lectures with 'PACE' inventor and genius Dan Hughes, who spent a full day with us teaching us how to help children with blocked trust relax and love again (PACE stands for playfulness, acceptance, curiosity and empathy, if you're wondering). Margot focused heavily on the new work of Stephen Porges, inventor of 'Polyvagal Theory', which shows us how the body reacts to threat and explains the secrets of our 'fight or flight' response. We learned to use paint, clay, puppets and sand trays to liberate children and allow them to reveal what was hurting them or holding them back. It felt like the most up-to-the-minute place to be, especially when we heard the government wanted every school to have a therapist on-site. We felt like an army being trained to fight against the newly named 'mental health crisis' and I guess we kind of were.

Overall it took almost four years to requalify and to chalk up enough 'therapeutic hours' of practice – and, just as I did, I gave birth to my first child. Suddenly my beautiful son Amiel was all I wanted to think about. He was born smiling and was and is such a joy in every way, but after a while the pressure to put to use what I had worked so hard to achieve made me feel I should emerge from maternity leave. Not to mention the loud roar of need from all of the depressed, scared and traumatised children at my school and in the wider world. Then, just as I opened my private practice . . .

The world was suddenly hit by the scariest threat in recent memory. Covid-19, an invisible killer, was racing round the world. We were trapped by laws and fear. We were told that leaving our homes could kill us. Seeing our friends or family was worse than outright murder. We were fearful of the things we had been doing our whole lives without ever previously thinking about them. The supermarket was an obstacle course of death and no one knew if they could trust the news, the government or the global response. It was scary for everyone and even worse for those who had traumatic childhoods.

Let me explain. If you had lived in a neglectful home with limited food, or lived with an eating disorder, seeing shelves empty of staples like pasta and eggs brought back deep-seated fear and panic. If you had parents you couldn't trust to care for you, you were retraumatised by the inability to trust those in charge. If you had spent years building a social life, a gym routine and a job to stave off your sadness and depression, or if you had made the choice to be self-employed and live far away in the countryside to have control over your own adult-hood in a way you did not in an overly controlling family, being at the mercy of this new, lonely and, for some, infantil-ising system all felt too much.

We lived in a life-threatened panic and chaos for nearly two years. It changed all of us and our anxiety levels forever.

The NHS reports that anxiety disorders affect around 5–10 per cent of the population in England. This includes conditions such as generalised anxiety disorder (GAD), social anxiety disorder, panic disorder and specific phobias. In the United States, the figures are even higher: the National Institute of Mental Health (NIMH) reports that anxiety disorders affect 31.1 per cent of adults at some point in their lives. According to data from the Mental Health Foundation, about 10 per cent of children and young people (aged five to sixteen) have a clinically diagnosable mental health disorder, and anxiety disorders are among the most common.

During the pandemic, children lived through worrying changes, deprived of their school schedule, but they were also deprived of friends, cousins and grandparents. They missed activities, teams and clubs. They missed being talked to, played with, cared for and checked on. They also missed out on having parents who knew what was happening and would happen next. It was scary and it didn't get better, causing the long-term and pervasive anxiety to set in.

It was very soon after that my practice changed. I was seeing almost exclusively anxious children. Too many of them to fit into my schedule and too many worried parents to start the phone calls to book them all in. My waiting list had a waiting list. I began to read, attend lectures and talk to practitioners in different fields about anything to do with anxiety.

And now I am going to share all I have learned with you.

How to use this book:

I recommend starting by considering whether your child's anxious feelings are new or whether they have always been an anxious kid. This will help you decide if looking at this as a short-term or long-term issue can help you start the process of supporting your child to feel better.

- If your child is newly anxious, start reading on page 53.
- If your child has always been anxious, start reading on page 90.
- If you are a naturally anxious parent, start reading on page 13.

Then think about your child's more specific issues. Do they struggle at bedtime? Worry themselves silly over exams? Have panic attacks? There will be a chapter for you!

In these pages you will discover specific advice for everything your child is going through, and a wealth of practical ideas to help you. The fundamental message is: anxiety erupts when safety is threatened. I will show you how to understand this threat and why your child is frightened. I will discuss symptoms and signs to watch out for. I will give real examples, though it is important to note that the case studies here are all composites with details changed to protect the privacy of the families I work with. I will explain how I helped that child and their family to conquer anxiety and reclaim their lives. I will provide ideas and scripts for right now and for the long term.

I will also advise you about when and how to speak to a doctor or your child's school and why that might be useful. I will outline the kinds of therapy or intervention that may be helpful and why.

My aim is to help you feel confident in supporting your family. Whether this is your first attempt to deal with your child's anxiety or you are a few months down the line, I will help you to feel better equipped and more relaxed while getting your child and your family life back.

Throughout the book you will see many 'Firework ideas'. These are quick strategies or flashes of inspiration that might just provide the bright spark you and your child have been waiting for.

In my practice, classroom or my own parenting I am at my most overwhelmed when I have exhausted all the ideas on my list. I love ideas. I will make sure you never run out of options. You will always have another plan to try.

I hope once you have used this book you can put it back on the shelf. If anxiety pops up again, remember this book and I will always be there waiting to help. Now let's get anxiety sorted!

Firework idea

The luckiest thing for our children is that they have us. We are the fortress between them and the scary world and we will work together to help them feel safe and restore their calm.

Part One:

Parental Anxiety

One

Help! I'm Anxious Just Reading This Book!

Anxiety is normal. It's the right and proper response when human beings – big or little – feel fear or believe they may be close to death. Now, *you* may know a burst balloon, a morning at playgroup or being put to bed in a nice safe cot doesn't warrant an explosion of fear and terror of death. The problem is that although *you* know it, your child doesn't.

While we're at it, you also know a business meeting, making a speech at a friend's wedding and creating a spreadsheet of your expenses are not truly terrifying and don't make you feel close to death. Yet you'll be first to admit all those situations bring on acute anxiety.

Let's break it down. If you mess up the meeting, you might lose your job. If you lose the job, you might lose your home. If you lose your home, you might be cold and hungry and you might get ill. You get the picture. Although one failed business meeting won't literally lead to your death, at a deep, primal level your brain picks up on the potential danger. The chemicals unleashed by your brain deliberately set up a pattern of anxiety so you will be on red alert to protect yourself against potential threats.

Anxiety is no accident. It's the brain's way of setting up a defence mechanism that will ultimately save your life.

It's that simple and that complicated.

To get the most benefit from this book, there are ten important things you need to understand. Once you get the hang of them, you'll be in the perfect position to calm your own anxiety and help your child in the fight against theirs.

1. Something or someone will have triggered your child's anxiety. It doesn't have to make sense to you, but that event or person has somehow set in motion a safety protocol in your child's brain.
2. Your child has no say over this at all. They may not realise what is happening to them or why. All they know is that they are scared and worried and their brain is pumping out cortisol, which increases their awareness of potential danger.
3. Your child is not doing or feeling this deliberately.
4. If you punish, scold or tell your child off for what you think is 'unreasonable' anxiety, it won't work. You'll make your child feel even less safe and even more anxious.
5. You cannot bribe your child not to feel anxiety. No reward is big enough to stop them feeling the fear. Trying to please you may lead them to try to mask their feelings, but they won't succeed.
6. The longer your child feels the fear, the worse the anxiety gets.

7. It can also spread to other unrelated things. Anxiety about attending birthday parties can expand into anxiety about play dates, school attendance or anything else as the amount of cortisol in their system increases. Everything in their life becomes scarier.
8. The opposite of anxiety is not CALM. The opposite of anxiety is SAFETY.
9. The way to soothe your anxious child is to increase their feeling of safety and connection.
10. YOU CAN DO THIS.

But before we start, a word on embarrassment, which is a feeling you might encounter when dealing with an anxious child in public . . .

Help! My child's anxiety is embarrassing the absolute bleep out of me!

Of course, you are embarrassed by your child's anxiety. You know they can't help it. I know they can't help it. But it doesn't change how you feel! The issue is that all the other children are happily trotting into school or tucking into a delicious tea or jumping for joy when their grandparents come over and greeting them enthusiastically. It feels as if it's only your child who finds school an impossible ordeal, will only eat plain white pasta with no sauce and stares fixedly at the wall when visitors arrive. You are embarrassed because you imagine other people are judging you and thinking there must be something lacking in your parenting. Your child's behaviour is showing you up, branding you an inadequate parent and everyone can clearly see your shortcomings.

It's tempting, when we feel ashamed and embarrassed, to take our humiliation out on the cause – our anxious child. Parents often shout at or punish their anxious children in public. They do it so no one will think they condone their child's strange behaviour. They want to signal clearly to onlookers that they are perfectly capable of instilling discipline in their children and make it obvious there is nothing wrong with the way they parent.

Although your embarrassment is natural – you wish your child would blend in and do the expected thing – don't be tempted to take your shame out on your anxious child. Don't try to project disapproval and tell your child off for the benefit of other people. Instead, focus on what your child needs – a feeling of safety and to know you are not judging them. They need to know you are in their corner and will support them.

If you must respond to onlookers, family or friends, say: 'X is feeling anxious about school/food/social occasions right now. It's very common for children of their age. We are working on supporting X through it.'

Permission to Leave

Remember, you can always take your child and go home. Nothing is forcing you to sit uncomfortably through a birthday party when your child is overwhelmed. They are not enjoying it. You are embarrassed. There's no point staying.

GO HOME! You can always try again another time. There will be more birthday parties.

Remember to be your child's advocate. If others ask, 'Why is he making such a fuss? It's only a plate of fish and chips!', answer, 'He has a sensitive and discerning palate. We think he's going to be Paul Hollywood when he grows up.' Laugh. Make light of their comments. Above all, enforce your child's feeling of safety by making it clear you are on his side and take no notice of what other people, even friends or family, say.

With that in mind, let's get to it . . .

Two

Help! I'm an Anxious Parent – How Do I Stop It Rubbing Off On My Child?

As parents, we have the ultimate responsibility of keeping another human being alive. If we mess up, the consequences are unthinkable. Nothing in our previous lives comes close to the pressure of being a parent.

Parenting is a relentless, 24-hour-a-day job usually done at the same time as working, managing a home and aiming to continue your other relationships. It comes at the cost of personal identity, sleep and time to do what you want to do. Is it any wonder we feel so anxious?

Being a parent changes you.

A 2010 study found that a mother's brain changes after giving birth. The amygdala, the brain's security centre, increases in size. The enlargement lasts for the rest of our lives. It ensures that mum will always be on red alert if there is a threat to her baby.

Amazingly, the same happens in adoptive parents too. A 2014 study showed one or both parents in adoptive families also see this growth in their amygdala!

With this heightened awareness of danger, our level of anxiety increases. None of this is relaxing.

Why are some parents more anxious than others?

All parents are novices. Even a second or third child is an entirely different individual from their older siblings. All parents are feeling their way and inexperienced at raising each new child. So why is it, when every mum and dad is in the same boat, some seem to sail through each new challenge and others flounder under the sheer weight of anxiety?

It's no surprise that your own upbringing influences the way you bring up your children. The model your parents gave you shapes the way you see yourself, how you form relationships and, of course, the way you view yourself as a parent. If your parents were calm, confident and capable – as well as present, kind and considerate – there's a very good chance you will parent in the same assured, positive and loving way. If, on the other hand, your parents were unavailable physically or emotionally, unkind, nervous, unreliable, unwell or in any way ill-equipped to deal with the challenges of parenting, they will have left you a legacy of doubt, fear and the key issue in this book – anxiety.

Attachment: the way a child forms a relationship with their parents

The way you form attachment will fall into one of four categories: secure, anxious, avoidant and disorganised. To work out the cause of you or your child's anxiety, it's helpful to identify your attachment category by examining your own upbringing and seeing which of the following models resonates with you. Remember, though, attachment is complicated. It is possible to have one kind of attachment to one parent and a completely different kind of attachment to the other.

Secure Attachment

A secure attachment means that the child believes that the parents will always love and care for them. The parent is reliable, sensible and loving.

If that describes your upbringing, you've won life's lottery. You're ahead of the game and so is your child. Secure attachment is exactly what you want to nurture in your own child.

Unfortunately, not all parents are lucky enough to have been brought up in this ideal environment. If secure attachment doesn't describe your upbringing, it will probably fall into one of the following categories. It is worth taking the time to think about which one most closely applies to you.

Anxious Attachment

An anxious attachment happens when a child doesn't know what to expect from their parents. Sometimes they are loving. Sometimes they meet the child's needs. But they are also critical, complicated and confusing. Their love is conditional and often withheld for no clear reason. The child knows their parent loves them and would probably help them if they needed assistance – but they cannot be sure. However hard they try, they can't predict how their parent will behave.

Obviously, this kind of parenting makes any child anxious. Experts say it can create love addicts. The child wants to be loved but doesn't know when the love they crave will be made available. The child needs love so deeply they will do anything in their limited power to secure it. This can lead to perfectionism: the child thinks that if their behaviour is flawless, they will be given the love they need. Children can also be clingy, loud or difficult to make sure they will get attention and love from their sometimes-unavailable parents.

If this description of anxious attachment resonates with you, you can see the way you were raised has set you up to be more anxious than other parents.

Avoidant Attachment

Avoidant attachment happens when a parent is cold and shut off. They meet some of the child's physical needs, but they are emotionally unavailable. They withhold physical affection and if the child expresses fear, anger or sadness, they ignore them or shout at them. Children of avoidant parents feel as if they are not allowed to have emotions. They push them away, which generates anxiety as it means they cannot own or trust their feelings.

Very sadly, if your parent left the family home or died, you will have had to navigate the gap left by an avoidant parent, even if their absence was unintentional.

If this description of avoidant attachment resonates with you, you will see why you find it difficult to trust your parenting instincts. You have been programmed to hide, ignore and mask your emotions. When you need to access them as a parent, you're lost and confused.

Disorganised Attachment

Disorganised attachment happens when a parent's choices, behaviour and personality are so unsafe and chaotic that the child is not adequately cared for. This upbringing might feature neglect or abuse, sexual or otherwise. The child must form an attachment to a parent who is not keeping them safe. They have no choice. The child loves the person who is doing them harm.

If this description of disorganised attachment resonates with you, I am so sorry you had such a tough time. It is no wonder you are anxious about your ability to be a parent. Don't worry, I've got your back. I'll help you through this.

It's not surprising so many of us are anxious.

Simon was a dad who got in touch because he was struggling with his teenage daughter. 'She told me to "f**k off"!' he said.

'Yes . . .?' I replied. 'And then what happened?'

'Nothing,' he said. 'She can't behave like this! She needs therapy!' He was booming down the phone.

'Well, what led her to be angry enough to be rude to you?'

'How should I know?'

'Umm, well, maybe we could work it out,' I coaxed. 'What was going on at the time? What were you talking about? Had you been arguing already?'

'Why do you need to know that?' he scoffed.

'Well, I guess I am trying to work out if you were riling each other deliberately? If she's angry without reason or if she's just a normal teenage girl pushing back and trying to find her place in your family, so she can work out where she ends and the rest of the world begins?'

'Oh,' he said and he began to sob. He sobbed throughout the conversation, discussing his fears for her and her siblings. Being their dad, it was his job to protect them, but he had no idea how to do it in a scary world. He had been so lucky with his kids and knew it. They were sailing through school. They had friends but he was terrified of being too lax, too strong, of missing his chance to mould them in the image he thought young women should fit into. He had had a complicated relationship with his own parents who had always been dismissive of him. Now, in adulthood, he saw them as little as possible, without severing ties. He was naturally anxious and, as a means to conceal this from his family, he had decided to pretend to be an authoritarian boss at home.

This was causing his children to push against his regime, generating in him a similar sensation to being dismissed by his own parents. The children also felt dismissed. He was ignoring their needs to try to maintain his own feeling of control over his family and his life.

Instead of strong-arming his daughter into therapy, he slipped happily into weekly therapeutic parenting support meetings himself.

Together we worked to understand the impact of his childhood on his parenting. He learned to listen to his feelings and stop masking his vulnerability. He worked on his self-esteem, learning to appreciate his best qualities. He began to realise which of his worries were significant and which a waste of his time.

Other Reasons You Might Be an Anxious Parent

- The body can feel the aftermath of highly stressful life events and turn them into a feeling of anxiety. Getting divorced, redundancy or the loss of a loved one can all leave us with fear and anxiety.
- Current affairs can increase anxiety. We feel powerless to influence them.
- Financial instability, ongoing work pressure or living with an emotionally or physically unstable family member can cause chronic stress.
- Being involved in a traumatic event such as a car accident or experiencing or witnessing abuse can have a lasting effect.
- Social factors such as isolation, difficult experiences with friends in childhood, moving and having to start again socially or feeling you can't meet the expectation of a social group can all contribute to later anxiety in adulthood.
- Substance abuse of drugs and alcohol exacerbate feelings of anxiety and worry that withdrawal will make life tougher.
- Excessive use of stimulants, including caffeine, can lead to increased anxiety.
- Living with a chronic illness, either your own or a loved one's, can have an impact on anxiety levels. This can be exacerbated by the additional needs that the condition may bring, the social exclusion that many people face, the

exhaustion brought on by the illness or care requirements, and the extra time needed for treatments or to compensate for physical restrictions.

- Fear of becoming unwell can plague people and cause anxiety.
- Poor sleep can drastically alter our mood and trigger anxiety.
- Those with depression, PTSD and other diagnosed or undiagnosed mental health disorders often have anxiety as a likely comorbidity.

Fundamentally, when we feel anxious as parents, for whatever reason, we too have lost a sense of security and safety – so now it's time to work to get it back!

What is the difference between daily and chronic anxiety?

Daily anxiety	Chronic anxiety
• Anxiety comes from a specific trigger in the moment. • When the stressor is removed or fixed, the anxiety subsides. • The anxiety feels proportional to how bad or worrying the problem is.	• The feeling of anxiety is almost permanent. It could be triggered by a real event or arise from nowhere. • Even when the problem or stressor has been sorted out or removed, the anxiety still feels very worrying.

- You may have symptoms like fast breathing, rashes, a racing heart, mild upset stomach or headaches but they feel like they have an end point that matches the end of the anxiety you are facing.
- Although you are worried or even panicked about something, you can still do the other things you need to do, like go to work, make a meal, tidy your house and organise important events.
- When given time to relax, talk to someone about your worries and implement coping strategies or self-care, the anxiety wanes.
- Although you might have bad days or could benefit from more formal support or counselling, you are able to relax sometimes and enjoy life when it is calmer.

- The anxiety feels all-consuming and doesn't match what is happening in real life. In other words, the consequences of what you are worrying about are minimal but the worry feels enormous.
- You may experience symptoms like headaches, short- or long-term stomach aches with IBS-like presentation, extended troubles with sleep, muscle tension and body aches. You may feel constantly frayed or overwhelmed or like everything is life or death/all or nothing.
- You feel like the anxiety is getting in the way of doing the things you need to do, like go to work, go to the supermarket or organise things in your life. You may have to take precautions to do things you used to do with ease, or you're unable to do tasks or go to certain places as they induce too much fear.
- The coping strategies you see others use seem too much to implement or don't feel like they would ever be enough. Or you've tried them and they don't work for you.
- You may have already sought help for your anxiety or you may feel that you cannot manage alone and will need additional support from a doctor or therapist to make a positive impact on your symptoms.

How can you calm down as an anxious parent?

1. Give Yourself a Break

Making the decision to buy this book to support your family shows that you are trying hard to be the parent you want to be. Parenting is tiring and worrying and the sheer effort required to do the right thing, sort out all the problems and keep everyone on the straight and narrow is exhausting. Parenting adds to the many things you are trying to negotiate successfully. I know it doesn't always feel that way, but you ARE doing a good job. Like most of the parents I speak to who are anxious, you are actually doing many things well enough, many very well indeed and some spectacularly. Let yourself release the worry that everything has to be perfect or that others are doing better.

There is no judge or jury for parenting. If you can manage to allow yourself to parent the way you want to, knowing your role is to try your best and have as much fun and as many good times with your family as possible, you can let yourself off the hook and liberate yourself from fear of failure.

2. Practise 'Self-care' – Whatever It Means for You

There is so much pressure to 'self-care' these days, but my feeling is that most people aren't sure what it means except maybe making time to work out. Maybe for some, a wet run on a dark October morning feels like self-care, but for many it would be more like self-punishment.

I want you to answer two questions:

- If you were your own kind parent, what would you do to care for you?
- Casting your mind back to when you were younger, before you had children, what kinds of things did you really enjoy?

I hope for the first question you will be thinking things like:

'I would put me to bed earlier.' 'I would make sure I eat more fruit.' 'I would only go running with a friend or in a parkrun because otherwise I lose myself in worrying thoughts.' 'I would tell myself it's OK to relax sometimes.' 'I would be less critical of myself.' 'I don't always need to rush.' 'I shouldn't care so much what others think.' 'I am allowed to like what I like.'

Or for the second question, you might be thinking:

'I used to love climbing trees.' 'I used to love sleeping in on a Sunday morning.' 'I used to love looking through catalogues.' 'I used to love playing with animals.' 'I used to love reading my favourite book over and over.' 'Sleepovers!' 'Teen magazines.' 'Being a goth!' 'Going to gigs.'

Use the ideas that popped into your head. Think about what you could add into your life that brings you the reassurance of being cared for by someone who loves and likes you. Write those ideas down in PEN in your diary or family calendar and start making them happen. If that means booking a baby-sitter or asking a friend for a favour so you can go and sit in the park for an hour with a coffee re-reading *Little House on the Prairie* or buying tickets to see McFly at a local festival, DO IT. Cancel only for a genuine emergency.

3. Practise Positive Self-talk

We all have an internal voice that hypes us up or tears us down. As we have seen, it is mostly scripted by the way our parents spoke to us. If your childhood was filled with validating positivity, that's wonderful, but 'gentle parenting' has only recently become popular, so most of us grew up with a greater or lesser degree of critical parenting.

The brain has a *negativity bias*. It takes at least five positive comments to cancel out one negative one. Unless your parents were constantly complimentary, your brain will have taken onboard the sense that there are many things you are not good at, you are less able than your siblings and friends and parts of your personality are downright repellent.

That voice might have been haunting you all your life. It has set you on a self-critical path. *Now is the time to free yourself.*

In Gestalt therapy, the therapist asks the client to record what their internal voice says about their appearance, skill level and personality. Listening back, they ask the client: 'Is that true? Is that helpful? What does believing these flawed ideas hold you back from?'

Change the way you speak to yourself. You can train your inner voice to be kinder and more supportive to yourself. When your brain says something like, 'Why would they want *you* there?', tell yourself, 'That's not kind or fair and I won't be my own bully.' Or: 'I am sure people will be happy to see me.'

Notice the way you talk to yourself about how you eat, look, think, behave and tell yourself to try again, speaking to yourself more gently, using kinder words.

Soon your brain will choose kind words automatically. You will programme yourself to speak as encouragingly to yourself as you would to others. You will notice a dramatic shift in your confidence when you are more compassionate and forgiving to yourself.

4. Change Your Life to Make It Safer

Which parts of your life make you anxious? Is it public places? Travelling? Going to the doctor? Socialising? Worrying that things will go wrong? How can you make them less fear-inducing?

Let's be practical! How can you be the master of your own life fortress? How can we help *you* feel safer?

Do you need a new doctor? Would having a break from certain friends or family members take off some pressure? Would looking for a new job give you a chance to be less worried about work? Do you need to save up to fix your back gate or get a camera for your house? What information would you need in advance about a social event to help you prepare for it?

Help yourself manage these issues as you would help your anxious child. Plan and prepare to provide the security you need to feel calmer.

One thing to note when you think about what might make you feel safer: if the answer leads you to restrict huge parts of your life, like not driving again or not leaving the house, it would indicate that your anxiety may need additional support from a GP or a therapist. Limiting your world will only increase cortisol production and the spread of the feeling of panic as more things become unsafe.

5. See Yourself the Way Your Children See You – and Fake It Till You Make It

I have often heard parents (usually mums) say they won't be in photos, even with their families, because of their overwhelming body anxiety. Sometimes, we hold ourselves back from connection and memories because of insecurities that the rest of the world and particularly our own children simply *do not see*.

Everything we do is copied and mirrored by our children. We are their building block for all behaviour. If we are worried about our weight, we give our children the clear message that weight is something they should worry about. Likewise, if we are scared of dogs, for example, our children will fear dogs, believing they are a threat.

So, it is important to ask yourself: what do I want my children to think about their bodies, dogs, exercise, their capabilities, and the safety of the world? Am I giving them the opposite message?

How do you talk about yourself? Could it be that you are saying either too much or too little about the things you wish your child knew about you? Think of the best parts of your character and story – you don't have to be serious. Jokes and funny stories will do the trick brilliantly. Remember, it's a good plan for you and your children to 'big yourself up' sometimes.

6. Help Your Brain Understand What's Happening

In so many situations, worry is caused by our brain misunderstanding how close we are to death. Sometimes it's easy to see why. Some examples:

- Hospitals make our brains fear we are close to death.
- Spiders – if poisonous – make our brains fear we are close to death.

- A break-in at home or work makes our brains fear we are close to death.

Other times, it's not so easy to understand why you're feeling this way. You might say, 'How can a social event/supermarket trip/worrying business meeting/making a phone call make my brain fear I am close to death?' The answer is: these situations trigger a reaction that might lead to a feeling of being left alone or being in danger. It might connect two false things to cause a reaction in your brain. Your job is to tell your brain the truth. You need to GIVE YOUR BRAIN A REALITY CHECK.

'Come on, brain, a meeting with Sally from the marketing team will not threaten my survival. The worst outcome will be a PowerPoint to review.'

'Come on brain, we are going to a familiar supermarket. We are not going at peak time. There won't be overwhelming crowds. We've been here many times before. My survival is not under threat.'

Talk your brain down from the ledge. This is not a good reason to panic. Give your brain a moment to get the message and regroup.

7. Teach Your Children to Take Risks Safely

The most anxious parents I see out and about are hovering over their children, fearful at all times they will hurt themselves.

Keeping your child safe is a frightening responsibility even if you are a qualified doctor, survivalist or police officer. The world feels scary to us, so we feel worried something might hurt our children. Understandably, parents try to protect their children by telling them to 'be careful'. Yet being constantly warned about some nameless danger makes some children more reckless and others more tentative. It doesn't make them any safer.

The key is to encourage your child to take measured risks in a safe way.

If they want to do something you think is dangerous – say they want to climb up steep stairs although they're only a baby or crawl over the top of the monkey bars at the park – instead of allowing your panic to dominate the situation, consider what skills or information your child, even at a young age, needs to accomplish their goal safely.

Instead of saying 'Be careful!', have a conversation about the safest way to climb a wall. Explain for now that they are just not big enough for abseiling, but that you will find a way for them to practise on something smaller and safer.

Help them slow down and focus on their hands and feet. Help them make their *own* survival strategy.

Instead of 'Be careful!' say, 'Look at your hands. Are you holding tightly enough? Look at your feet. Have you thought about what to do about it being slippery below you?'

This method works for all life challenges. Plan in advance, slow down and make the next move carefully.

8. Prioritise Sleep

Sleep could be the crucial ingredient to reducing your anxiety. Doctors treating patients with mental health issues coupled with either exhaustion or insomnia will say treating the sleep issue first is guaranteed to have a positive effect on the mental health disorder.

On average, adults over twenty-six need between seven and nine hours of sleep per night to function at their best. Parenting, however, is often interspersed with disturbed sleep.

Whether you have a teething two-year-old or a wakeful six-year-old, careful 'sleep hygiene' with a few cheeky naps thrown in for you can make all the difference.

If you are *sleep-deprived* (i.e. you want to sleep but cannot because you do not have adequate opportunity), try to implement the following changes in the short term:

- Nap, as often as you can.
- Try making the whole family's bedtime earlier. If your child usually wakes up at midnight, aim to have had a few hours' sleep before then.
- Try getting yourself and your family outside into nature daily to boost your circadian rhythm.

And in the long term:

- Try to increase time in bed even by a small amount. Switch off your smartphone. Don't scroll when you could sleep.
- Aim to be consistent with sleep to help decrease your sleep debt. Keep bedtime at a regular earlier time six days a week for at least a month.
- If you still feel sleepy and anxious, make an appointment to discuss your sleep deprivation with a doctor.

If you are suffering from *insomnia* (i.e. you want to sleep and have adequate opportunity to do so, but can't):

- Set an alarm to wake yourself at the same time every day even if you are tired.
- Avoid napping.
- Get up and out of bed straight away – no pushing the snooze button.
- Open the curtains or window or get outside early. Light in your eyes earlier in the day can help set up your circadian rhythm, which will help you fall asleep at night.
- Only get into bed when you are drowsy.
- Only use your bedroom for sleep, sex and getting dressed. ALL other activities including working, reading, watching TV and even prayer or meditation should be done somewhere else to condition the feeling that bedrooms are for sleeping.

- If you do not fall asleep within fifteen minutes, get out of bed however hard it is and get back in when you feel drowsy again.
- Avoid caffeine after 2 p.m.
- Avoid alcohol in the evening as it makes us sleep more easily but wake up earlier.

Firework idea

Try stopping your night-time TV viewing thirty minutes earlier. An extra thirty minutes of sleep can make you feel better for all sixteen waking hours of the next day!

9. Invest in Relationships

I see so many parents affected by loneliness due to the number of hours in the day they are either alone, or doing things that make them feel alone.

Choose the friends that make you feel happiest and make it a *rule* to see each other or book in time for a phone call once a month.

Apps like Garden or Be Friends have been designed to remind you to check in on your friends and make sure they check in on you too!

Ask someone you like but don't know well over for coffee or a plate of simple food you feel confident preparing. The act of giving hospitality, provided you keep it simple, can lessen loneliness.

10. Don't Be Afraid to Work on Yourself

When you read the list of reasons for adult anxiety or the information on attachment (see pages 18 to 26), did one or more stand out for you? Do you think looking into those areas with a counsellor, psychotherapist or doctor would help you feel more in control of your life? You do not need to be in a crisis to work on yourself with a professional to get better and find life easier.

Therapy is often not what people expect. People feel worried therapy will expose them or unhinge them. The therapist, if trained and experienced, will guide you and be guided by you. Their expertise and kindness will be used to help you learn about yourself and your history and support you to make you feel less anxious and more content with your life.

Therapy or counselling can help you achieve the feeling of safety you are hoping to offer your children because it helps you explore your personality, thoughts and feelings in a secure, caring environment.

When should you ask for help from a professional and what kind of help is right for you?

We've all heard 'It's OK not to be OK,' but I always add, 'You don't have to stay that way!'

If you are too anxious to leave your home, you cannot do the things on your to-do list because your anxiety holds you back or you are so overwhelmed that you are showing anger to your children in a way that makes you uncomfortable, it may be time to look for additional support for your mental health.

Here are some options:

Personal Therapy

Look for a therapist in your local area who is qualified and registered with a therapeutic body like UKCP, BACP or BAPT to make sure the therapist you see has the endorsement of a professional group.

Each of the therapeutic bodies has a directory of practitioners (search 'UKCP directory' or 'BACP directory', etc.). Use the filters to hone in on the kind of therapy you're looking for – e.g. whether you want it online or in person, the locality, whether you want a male or female practitioner and so on. You can also search for a specific type of therapist by googling 'art therapist directory' or 'counselling directory', for example. Try to find two or three therapists that appeal to you. Read their listings and see if you respond to the way they express themselves. See if they have experience with anxiety as well as any of the other things in your life that could have had an impact on you. Then get in contact with those you feel good about and see if they have availability for you.

If you worry about the price of therapy, some therapists may have reduced rates for certain groups of people.

The aim is to find someone in your price bracket who is kind, available and supportive who will work to help you feel better.

Cognitive Behavioural Therapy (CBT)

CBT works to help a person stop doing certain behaviours that make their life less positive. Some of the coping strategies that result from anxiety may be hurting us in the long run and we can use the practical methods and structure taught to us by a CBT therapist to help us stop doing those things.

CBT can also help to work out which negative messages we are sending ourselves and help us to see the world differently. It can help us break anxious thought patterns for good.

Mindfulness-Based Stress Reduction (MBSR)

MBSR teaches mindfulness meditation to help individuals become more aware of their thoughts and feelings in the present moment, reducing anxiety and improving overall wellbeing.

Other mindfulness or meditation practices can also help. There are also lots of apps now that can support meditation and mindfulness practice at home. Try Headspace, Insight Timer or Smiling Mind.

Group Therapy

Group therapy helps people find support with others who are struggling. It can help us feel connected to others and gives us regular contact with fellow participants in a supportive environment. Having other people as part of your therapeutic process can help us take responsibility for ourselves. It is also usually a lot cheaper than personal therapy.

Google 'group therapy for parents'. You can add 'near me' or 'online' depending on what you are looking for.

Support Groups

Support groups are similar to group therapy and should be run or managed by someone with some therapeutic or medical expertise. The difference is that a support group is likely to have a more casual, dip-in nature and the group may change regularly, whereas a therapy group would usually be formed of about eight participants and then continue with the same people at the same time each week or month for a set amount of time.

Groups could also be set up to help with a specific purpose, such as breastfeeding, parenting children with ASD or LGBTQIA+ child support.

Psychiatric Services

Psychiatric services are available for parents who would like medicine to support their mental health. In the UK, you can go to your GP and ask for a referral to see a psychiatrist who will listen to your symptoms and history. The psychiatrist may need to do blood tests or ask for information about any other medication you take to then decide which psychiatric medication would work for you.

Many adults and children need medication to live their happiest lives. Only a few years ago, people would have been embarrassed to say they were having therapy. I think soon most people will proudly talk about the medication they take that makes their life more manageable.

Online Therapy

Since 2020, online therapy has become the norm. If trying to fit therapy into your life is complicated – for example if you need to organise childcare or travel – online therapy can make life simpler, as you can have your session while your kids sleep or are at school, or you are away from your own home. Use the normal therapeutic directories like UKCP and BACP – put in a preference for online therapy and find highly qualified therapists providing their services either in or out of working hours.

Couples Therapy

A huge feeling of security can be restored when we believe our partner is in this with us. Finding a couple's therapist online or in person can calm the soul of both you and your partner, and re-centre your family as both of you are investing in the process.

You cannot force your partner to go to therapy with you. But it may persuade them if you highlight that you are missing being with them, feel like you are rarely on the same page and that you are ready to work out how to be better now rather than separate later.

Parenting Support Courses

Local councils can offer both short and long parenting courses. You should be able to access services like:

- Home start: perinatal mental health support.
- CRY-SIS helpline: support for parents with crying and sleepless babies.
- Family Links: the parenting puzzle free online programme.
- Empowering Parent Empowering Communities (EPEC)
- Resilience tutoring for parents.
- Parent GYM: free parenting skills training offered by local boroughs, often through schools.

- Strengthening Families, Strengthening Communities (SFSC) – reducing parental conflict.

Search for parenting courses on your local council website or search for similar private parenting courses.

Life Coaching/Mentoring

Life coaching can provide very personal and practical support. Like finding a personal trainer for your physical health, coaching can help by bringing a person with experience into your life to support you in maintaining the structures and routines that are necessary to help you function at your best.

Parent Support Phone Calls

A service I offer, which many other therapists do too, is a parent support phone call. Whether you are worried about your child or yourself, the call can be an opportunity to think through what you have been doing and see if there are any firework ideas or small changes we can come up with to support you and your family.

EFT (Emotional Freedom Technique) Tapping

If the idea of sitting quietly with your thoughts fills you with dread but calm is what you seek, consider learning about

EFT tapping through online videos or a short online training course.

Tapping uses Eastern medicine's meridian lines to show you where to tap on your body to give it the signal that you are safe. Tapping has a set system that can be done relatively quickly and can be fitted into our busiest days to help us calm down.

Important: If you ever feel like hurting yourself or think that you cannot continue feeling the way you do, contact your GP immediately, go to a walk-in A&E or contact a crisis team in your local area.

Let's talk about postnatal anxiety and depression

People often talk about postnatal depression (PPD), but rarely discuss postnatal anxiety (PPA), which is when the change in hormones after having a baby leads to acute and excessive anxiety.

Similarly to PPD, it usually occurs within the first six weeks after birth, but it can happen any time before your child's first birthday and still be considered PPA. If unchecked or ignored, it could continue to affect a person for years.

How to identify it:

- Worrying excessively, particularly about the safety or health of the baby, to the point at which you cannot do the things you need to do.
- Feeling extremely irritable or angry all the time.
- Restlessness. Difficulty relaxing or feeling constantly 'on edge'.
- Not being able to sleep due to anxiety, even when the baby is calm or asleep.
- Regularly experiencing the physical symptoms that can be attributed to anxiety such as headaches, nausea, dizziness, heart palpitations or muscle tension.
- Having fast-paced, overwhelming thoughts that feel as if you cannot control them.
- Fear of being alone, particularly if left with the baby or child. Or feeling panicky when you have to leave the baby even for a short time.
- Panic attacks.
- A clear increase or decrease in appetite.
- Feeling overwhelmed, particularly making decisions or managing responsibilities related to the baby.
- Hypervigilance.
- Avoidance or isolation.

If you recognise these signs in yourself or someone you know, it's important to take action. Here are steps you can take:

- Notice your feelings are abnormal to you. Notice that they are different or more extreme compared to the way you usually experience stress.
- Tell someone: a partner, parent or friend.
- Visit a GP or your gynaecologist.
- Consider finding a therapist or look into any of the other support options listed above.
- Rest and sleep if you can and as much as you can.
- Go outside at least once a day.
- Eat well and aim to feel full as you recover.
- Find relaxing moments and avoid adding more stressful things to your list.
- Find a trusted and experienced person to consult when you have questions about your baby.
- After you have identified you may have PPA, read about it and try to understand it is very common and treatable.
- Set small goals like getting to the end of each day safely.
- Do the easiest things to care for yourself and the baby.
- Give yourself kindness. Having a baby is very, very hard and your body is not helping you.
- Be proactive in asking for help.

If this is happening to you, I am very sorry. It must be very hard and you do not deserve it. Please reach out to someone – a GP, a therapist online or near you, or a charity such as PANDAS Foundation or Mind UK – and prioritise yourself and your baby until you feel better.

Firework idea

One of the fastest ways to calm the adult body is to listen to your body's needs as they happen. As a parent, we often delay going to the loo, eating, drinking or sitting down, which promotes a feeling that it is OK to ignore our needs. This can keep us in a panic mode as our body might think we aren't popping to the loo because we are being chased or under threat. If we aim to meet our need as soon as it comes up, or if we tell ourselves we are safe and we'll do it as soon as we can, our body will relax, as it will know we are safe and just busy changing a nappy.

Part Two:
Helping an Anxious Child

Three

Help! My Child is Suddenly Anxious

Some parents are lucky; their child arrives in this world with an innate calmness and belief that all will be OK. Let's call this baby Max. Chilled Max doesn't dissolve into inconsolable tears if you give him the orange cup instead of the purple. He recovers quickly from a bump on the knee and copes with change easily. Even the potential ordeal of going to a new nursery or school is a breeze for this relaxed chap. The rest of us look on longingly.

Naturally, Max's parents feel fantastic. They are used to a cheerful, carefree child. His emotional stability reflects positively on their parenting. His calmness relaxes them and makes them feel calm in return. They have never had to worry about building up Max's defences. They've never had to run through the day in their minds before it even happens, trying to pre-empt the events that might unsettle him.

Then, suddenly, Max starts showing obvious signs of anxiety. His parents are surprised. His anxiety manifests as a fear that sticks. They try making light of it, but can't seem to dislodge it. His parents become acutely worried. They doubt themselves. They barely recognise the Max they know and love. They feel out of their depth and desperate, as if Max's anxiety is going to capsize their family.

Max was six when his parents contacted me. They talked about their shock at the changes in their previously contented, well-settled child. They explained nothing had changed. They simply couldn't work out what had agitated and distressed their happy little boy.

We arranged for me to meet him. We played, painted and talked. It was a lovely session with a happy, well-regulated boy. I couldn't immediately pinpoint the problem and was beginning to worry that I wouldn't be able to help the family. Then, as we got up to leave, Max turned to me and said, 'You've got a lot of story books. You'd better lock those up at night.' He said it with a friendly face and a manner that looked as if he thought his advice was excellent.

He believed intensely that my books were under threat of being stolen. Why? I stopped walking him out and said, 'Thank you for your advice . . . Why do you think I should lock up my books?'

'Well, you have to watch out for the book bandits,' he replied.

'Remind me about those book bandits . . . I think I've forgotten,' I said with a friendly smile.

'Umm . . . I don't really like to talk about it, but I've seen the video at school of the book bandits who stole all our reading books.'

It turned out that at his lovely, friendly local school, they had tried to engage the children with a topic excitingly named

'The Book Bandits Strike'. It required the children to write and read clues and reports about their stolen books to win them back at the end of the week. Extra drama was supplied by a video of the class teacher and teaching assistant dressed in Zorro outfits running around the school. The clip of them jumping on the tables in the lunch hall and crawling through the school library with a copy of *Harry Potter* in their teeth was meant to be a humorous and light-hearted way to inspire the children to work hard.

For Max, however, it was a violation of his safe place. He didn't find the Book Bandits funny in the least. To him they were terribly, shockingly scary. The feeling that the school could be entered and pillaged at any time caused Max to be hypervigilant and terrified to attend. As it seemed the other children hadn't felt the same and the books were returned by Friday, the little boy kept the feeling to himself.

What happens when your child has anxiety

Anxiety occurs when an initial experience violates our feeling of safety and triggers our fight or flight system to release adrenaline and make us do what we can to get us to safety.

Watching the video of the Bandits pilfering their books, Max knew that he wasn't in immediate danger, as they'd already left the building. But the possibility of their return, or any other trespasser breaking in, told his brain and body to stay on red alert. The fact that the other children thought it was funny made his feelings even more confusing. At home, as most children do, Max said his day had been 'fine'. His parents didn't realise their boy had changed until he started having terrible nightmares, a constant tummy ache, said he didn't want to go back to school a few weeks later and refused point blank to stay after school for clubs he had always loved.

Max couldn't just 'snap out of it'.

Max's sudden-onset anxiety was brought on by a violation of his feeling of safety. His body was now consistently pumping a small amount of extra cortisol into its system to make sure Max was on red alert if a school invasion happened again. The Book Bandits activated a system called the hypothalamic-pituitary-adrenal (HPA) axis, which continually sends signals and chemicals to keep us worried – but not worried enough to act – about a possible threat. This can elicit what we more commonly call the 'fight, flight, freeze, fawn response', leading to these drastically different stress responses that we see in children. As the cortisol continues to drip into our system, we feel more and more nervous about everything and completely lose our feeling of safety and control.

How do you know if your child has sudden-onset anxiety?

The symptoms we most commonly see in children who are suddenly anxious are:

- Being or acting scared.
- Wanting to stay at home.
- Separation anxiety.
- Stomach aches.
- Headaches.
- Changes in eating – either overeating or not feeling hungry.
- Changes in sleep – overnight wake-ups, bad dreams, wanting to sleep near you, finding it hard to fall asleep.
- Finding things that are usually easy very difficult.
- Wanting more physical contact.
- Withdrawing.
- Skin picking.
- Hair pulling.
- Asking lots of extra questions about where you are going or who will be there.
- Looking worried or pale.
- Acting out with siblings or younger children, e.g. hitting, not wanting to share or being bossy.
- Not wanting to go to places they usually go, like clubs, activities or friends' houses.
- Going to the loo more frequently, accidents from children who have been potty trained for a while, or holding in wee and poo in an irregular way.
- Crying more frequently.
- Finding it difficult to concentrate.

Let's talk about hypervigilance

When children become 'hypervigilant', they effectively turn into their own security guard. Imagine how exhausting it must be surviving the school day, attending after-school gymnastics and changing into your pyjamas while doing your very best to subject every noise, person and place you encounter to a personal security patrol. Children don't choose to be hypervigilant. The behaviour is a subconscious response to fears and worries about school-life. It's the body's way of trying to keep itself safe.

If your child is hypervigilant, you will notice them:

- Jumping at loud noises.
- Flicking their head or body round at speed to check who has come in the door.
- Not wanting to be left alone.
- Not blinking regularly.
- Not wanting to sit with their back to the door.
- Asking for extremely detailed information about daily plans in what feels like a forensic way.
- Checking doors and windows.
- Asking the same questions repeatedly even though you have already given them the answers.

Parents can find managing a hypervigilant child exhausting. Their need to arm themselves with information and be one step ahead feels impossible to support. Furthermore, being close to someone who is in survival mode, scanning and checking and unable to relax, makes our own adult bodies and brains feel unsafe. We start to wonder if we are missing a dangerous threat our child can see. We become more and more uncomfortable under the weight of their fears and alert to the possibility that we are in danger too.

Remember: Symptoms Don't Always Appear Immediately

Some children will start to show symptoms immediately making it much easier to pinpoint the security breach in their system. For example, if your child went to Grandad's house and watched a film that scared them:

- They may be scared at pick-up.
- They may be scared at bedtime that night.
- They may identify their fear the next time they go to Grandad's.

However, sometimes it is not so obvious. If your child's system takes longer to feel the cortisol or they have been distracted – for example, leaving Grandad's and going straight to a party then having a full week of school and activities – the other more enjoyable chemicals that our body makes, like oxytocin, dopamine, serotonin and endorphins, may cover the cortisol enough for the child to have minimal symptoms until the cortisol builds up or the good feelings die down – often several days later.

Remember, too, that symptoms can grow more pronounced after the event that has triggered it. Over time, the minimal overproduction of cortisol can exacerbate anxiety and symptoms become more visible and acute. Some parents find that the symptoms seem to have popped up overnight many weeks after the triggering event and that may be to do with the extended exposure to more cortisol.

Anxiety doesn't have to be logical to be real

Our job is to work to restore the feeling of safety or connection that our child instinctively feels has been taken away, whether or not we know the exact cause and regardless of whether the anxiety makes logical sense to us. Our brains make decisions about our safety based on half-formed sensations using the hippocampus, a part of the brain in charge of memory but also dreams. Your child's safety gauge adds up emotions, bits of pictures and things sensed but not necessarily real. This is why our children's anxieties (and our own) don't make sense; they are not grounded in fact. Just as you can wake up from a dream angry or worried even though nothing in the dream actually happened, anxiety can be caused in the same complicated way.

A child can be told that a character cannot climb out of the TV, but their brain and body are not sure.

A child can be told that you won't ever leave them, but when you walk off into the distance at nursery, their brain and body are not sure.

How to help: first steps

We need to try to identify the original offending experience, push it out of our child's mind and put things in place emotionally and physically to let them know their safety has been restored. We need them to know they can relax, stand down their 'internal artillery' and carry on enjoying life and doing all the things they love to do.

Step One: Identify the Catalyst

As soon as you have noticed the symptoms of anxiety or hypervigilance in your child, it's time to start thinking about the catalyst (cause).

Have any major changes happened in your family's world in the last six months to a year? For example, have you experienced any of the following?

- Have you had a baby?
- Have you moved house?
- Have you been unwell or had an unwell family member?
- Has anyone you know died?
- Has your child started or moved school?
- Has there been a separation or divorce in your family?
- Have you had trouble conceiving or had pregnancy complications or loss?
- Has your child had a close friend leave school or move classes?
- Has a pet died?
- Have you been at home less than usual?
- Have you been very worried about something at work or at home?
- Has your child had a sleepover or a play date that may have been irregular or worrying?
- Has your child had a worrying social experience, been bullied or hurt at school, been left out or upset during school or an after-school club?
- Has your child been doing any exams or rigorous testing at school?
- Has your child watched or read anything unusual?
- Was there anything they mentioned in the last month or so that didn't get enough time to be explored or properly resolved?

If the answer to any of the above questions is 'Yes', you will find more advice on how to deal with all these anxieties later in the book. However, sometimes there is no obvious cause for your child's anxiety. Whether you have pinpointed the reason or not, the next step is the same: you need to talk to your child to try to find out more about their specific fears and help them manage their feelings.

Let's talk about the window of tolerance

First of all, what is a window of tolerance? The idea behind this is that depending on what has been going on for us – i.e. how tired, stressed, sad or hungry we are – we will be able to tolerate different things to different levels. When we are inside our window of tolerance, we can manage all that we come up against. However, when we are overwhelmed, having a bad day, or are worrying about something, you will find it takes less to rile you up, make you cry or make you check out of the situation.

For example, if we are stressed as we wake up because our alarm didn't go off, then the washing in the dryer isn't dry, then the bus is late, we may have already exited our window before we even finish school drop-off.

If we are overwhelmed like this, we may end up coming out in a heightened way from our window, which is called **hyperarousal**. If we are hyperaroused, we may feel angry, anxious or out of control. It can trigger our fight or flight response.

If we are so overwhelmed that we feel it is all too much and we want to retreat from the world, it is as if we are leaving our window of tolerance through the bottom, as our chemical arousal drops to give us the feeling of wanting to step back from the world. We call this **hypoarousal**. We may feel numb, frozen, checked out, unable to concentrate, spacy.

If, after a bad morning, you were hyperaroused, you may find yourself rushing panicked down the high street shouting, 'We're going to be late – for goodness' sake don't look at that dog and don't stop to smell those blinking flowers!'

If you were hypoaroused, you might quietly capitulate and say, 'We're late but who cares, it doesn't matter anyway.' Then you may be so preoccupied with your own thoughts and busy separating yourself from the guilt of messing up you and your child's day that you hardly even remember to say goodbye. Then, as if by magic, you are back at home, not even sure which route you took.

Some days, a child spilling their glass of water all over their sibling will lead to rage, a hyperarousal response. Other days it will just lead to laughter. This indicates that we are doing better, allowing us to have a larger window of tolerance.

We can use this knowledge of our window of tolerance and a guess about how big our child's window is to decide when to have our conversation about their anxiety.

Step Two: Talk to Your Child About Their Anxiety

Whether or not you've managed to identify the catalyst for your child's anxiety, either way the next step is to prepare yourself for a quick but deep chat with your child.

Consider beforehand that you will need space in your window of tolerance (see above) to manage them if they reveal something sad, surprising or scary. So think about the following before you embark on your conversation:

- Have your chat earlier in the day when neither of you are overtired. Ensure you also give yourself a window of at least two hours before bedtime so that they have time to calm down again if something big comes up.
- Make sure you both aren't hungry when you sit down to chat. You could even give them something crunchy like crisps to nibble on when you talk, as chewing crunchy things can let the body know it is safe; your child will feel like they are grazing calmly like a cow in a field rather than running like an antelope chased by a lion in a savannah.
- Set up the conversation to take place in a structured time frame: a walk round the block, a drive to an activity, a breakfast picnic in the park. When you start the conversation, you can say, 'I just wanted to chat for a few minutes about something I've been wondering about,' so your child knows this will have an end and *you* know you only have a finite time you need to hold it together.

- Aim to have the conversation with one child at a time. Even if you will need to talk to more than one child about something, aim to give them each time to talk about it separately. They may have a different response, which might make the other feel misunderstood or as if their feelings are wrong.
- Consider having a side-by-side rather than face-to-face conversation – walking next to each other, driving with them in the back, or sitting next to each other on a bench or at a table at a café. This can take off the pressure they may feel to reveal their soul while being stared at. It can help children talk more and feel less self-conscious. This is particularly useful for teenagers.
- Give opportunities for safe and appropriate touch through-out. You can hold hands, start and or end with a hug, stroke their back or head if they like it. You could give them inter-mittent hand squeezes or pats as you go.

Now, what should you say?

The aim of the conversation is to achieve three things:

1. To find out what the issue might be and where it stems from.
2. To think of practical solutions together while staying calm.
3. To show our children we can manage the situation and the feelings they have around it.

Here are some examples:

Beth is a seven-year-old child who is upset about friends and school.

> Parent: I just wanted to chat for a few minutes about something I've been wondering about. I've noticed that for the past few weeks you have seemed a little worried / scared / stressed out / funny and I've been thinking about what might be going on.
>
> *[At this point, you can wait and even count ten seconds in your head. That might be enough to start the conversation.]*
>
> Beth: Yeah, you're right. I have been feeling funny.
>
> Parent: Any idea what's set that off?
>
> *[Wait again. You are aiming to keep your face looking serious but positive. You may need to breathe more deeply than usual to manage the unknown elements of this conversation. Remember, you are looking to begin classifying the kind of anxiety they are struggling with and what primal fear it triggers. Then you can put a clear plan in place to stop the possibility that the fear will happen again, so that your child and their body understand all is well.]*
>
> Beth: My friends have been leaving me out and I have been worried I won't have anyone to play with.
>
> *[This child is showing signs of social anxiety. We know that the amygdala (the alarm centre of the brain) is triggered by*

social separation to believe we are in danger – maybe because historically, humans have survived better in packs; maybe because alone we would find it harder to get resources or our needs met. Or maybe it's because the brain knows that without social interaction, we will become lonely, which can lead to a depression of the chemicals in our system, making us feel sad and low and even more excluded. Whatever the reason, social anxiety can cause our bodies to feel very unprotected.]

Beth: For the last two weeks, it's been much harder to play as we have now moved to the big playground and my friend mostly wants to play basketball.

[I know, lots of children are not this articulate or clear, but what we are trying to find out is the whens and wheres and what makes the anxiety worse. If you haven't worked it out yet, you can now ask:]

Parent: What do you think your biggest fear is in this situation? / Which part of that feels the most difficult?

Beth: I'm scared no one will play with me / I don't know what to do during break time / I don't know how to sort it out.

Parent: Gosh, I hear that you are feeling lonely at school and that you feel like you don't have ideas for the playground to make it fun again. Is that right?

[Here we summarise to check we have understood. The child will say yes, or correct you if you've got it wrong.]

Parent: Well, you are clever, I am clever. I'm sure we can come up with a plan to sort this out. Do you have any ideas?

[Wait and let the child think first. All the ideas they say should be received positively. For example, if a child says, 'I should punch all my friends!', you might respond, 'Woah, you are really angry with them, and so am I. But I think when we calm down, we can look at this again and see if we can come up with another plan, as I don't want you to get in trouble because they aren't being nice to you.' If they don't have any ideas, you can say:]

Parent: It's hard to come up with ideas, I'll suggest some and if there are any you like, we can do them. How about . . .

You then come up with a few options. They might include things like:

1. We talk to your teacher about options at lunchtime.
2. We have play dates with other kids in your class.
3. We practise talking to your friends and explaining how you feel.
4. We draw a map of the playground and plan out each day what you think you want to do. Then you can do it and see which friends want to join in.

Listen to their response. If they don't like your ideas, think of more. If you are sure you need to speak to the teacher, say,

'Well, the first thing I'm going to do is mention it to your teacher. You can come with me or tell them yourself. Can you decide what else we do next?' Then give your options.

Do the things you've agreed to do from your list then set a time to come back to them and remember to talk about it again.

In making a plan and executing it, the end may come very quickly. It may solve the problem and calm the body.

Ridian, age nine, has been worrying about his grandma, who is in hospital.

Ridian: I have been thinking about Nanny a lot since she went into the hospital last week.

[This child is already showing a few possible worries here – we could be seeing fear of change, fear of death and/or health anxiety. These fears about change in their life or losing access to people they love can be some of the scariest. The child may be fearful of a loss of connection with that person, nervous that a parent will be around less as they may have to look after the other family member, or they may have been pushed to wonder about a time when you or a co-parent may be ill, unavailable or gone. Proximity to illness and death scares our body as it cannot work out by itself that if someone else is ill then we won't naturally catch it and get ill ourselves.]

Parent: How long have you felt that way? / When do you notice your worry the most?

Ridian: I find myself mostly worrying about Nanny in bed and when I am alone. Sometimes I can't concentrate at school because I am thinking about whether something might happen to her.

Parent: What do you think your biggest fear is in this situation? / What do you think the hardest part of that is?

[Listen to their response and repeat it back to them to make sure you've understood. Acknowledge the strength of their fear, for example:]

Parent: Oh my love, I can hear that that is very scary and nervous-making. No wonder you have been worried.

[What you say next depends on how ill the grandparent is. If the grandparent is unlikely to die, you could say:]

Parent: I have also been worried about Nanny and wondering if she will be OK. Maybe we haven't given you enough information about what is going on. This is what we know at the moment *[insert factual but not additionally worrying information about the situation here]*. The most important thing is that she is being looked after by clever doctors and they have said that she should get better and I am going to help her get home as soon as possible. Do you have any other questions?

[If the grandparent is likely to die, you could say:]

Parent: I have also been worried about Nanny and wondering if she will be OK. Maybe we haven't given you enough information about what is going on with her and it is possible that at some point we will have more sad news, but for now, this is what we know *[insert factual but not additionally worrying information about the situation here]*.

[Now put in as many easy-to-understand safety walls as you can. The information we are trying to get across here is:

- *You cannot catch what they have.*
- *Clever doctors are managing it.*
- *You will always be looked after no matter what.*
- *Whatever happens, we will get through it together.*

So, tell your child these things clearly while making physical contact to help the body regulate and feel managed:]

Parent: As you know, you and I cannot catch what Nanny has, so although she is unwell, we will be well enough to look after her and help her while she is sick. I trust the doctors to help her [or help her manage this difficult part well] and I know they are doing all they can. I want you to know that no matter what happens, we will always be here for you, look after you and make sure you have exactly what you need. Whatever happens, we are a strong team and we will get through it together. Do you have any questions?

Offer space for questions and answer what you can. If a question comes up that you don't know the answer to, tell your child you will think about it and get back to them. If they haven't got any questions or say they don't know, let them know they can come back and ask you at any time and you will answer as soon as you can.

You can also ask them what they think will help them manage their worries. Let them think of options. If it's not possible for them to fit into the plans for the ill family member, such as a hospital visit, explain why that is. Say you understand it might feel hard not to be able to do what you want, then offer something else, like writing a letter or doing a video call if appropriate.

After this very sad and difficult conversation, imagine your job is now to wrap your child up like a tiny baby in a warm blanket. It doesn't have to be literal – you can do other things like check in on them more, surprise them with nice things, or draw them a lovely warm bath. Show them in your presence and care how loved and looked after they are.

Sometimes, fears are more abstract. Khadija, age eight, is worried about something scary.

> Khadija: My friends have been talking about a killer that was in a movie they watched on Halloween. Even though I wasn't there, it's getting stuck in my head.

> [*This sort of fear, based on something not real, can surprise or blindside parents. Their child has been invaded by something that cannot actually be a danger, but knowing what to do*

next about a fear or phobia, whether real or pretend, can be so hard. The child in this case also has the power of their own brain working against them. Their brain is telling them they are in danger and adding images, ideas and chemicals to the mix to make it even more inescapable.]

Parent: Wow, that sounds really difficult, I'm sorry you have been managing that alone. I'm pleased you have told me now.

[This may be a good point to stop what you're doing and look at your child, hold hands or make physical contact. If driving, wait until it is safe and give them a clear look in the rear mirror so they can see you are really listening and here to connect and help with these feelings. In letting them know we are here and available, the body will immediately feel even a tiny bit safer as they are no longer fighting this fear alone.]

Parent: How long have you felt that way? / When do you notice your worry the most?

[Here we are gathering information without planting additional fears or assuming we understand how they feel.]

Khadija: Since Halloween, they've played this game at lunch where one is the killer and we all have to hide. It makes me feel weird and then I've been thinking of him and I think he's coming to get me.

Parent: What do you think your biggest fear is in this situation? / Which part of that feels the most difficult?

Khadija: I'm scared he's coming to get me / I don't like playing the game but I feel I can't stop them.

Parent: Oh, poor you, it sounds like it's been rough the last few weeks, having joined in with something scary and then thinking about it all the time. You know I have to tell you [*big smile on your face and calm eyes*] in all my years on this earth I have never met a killer on the loose and you know I would never let anyone unsafe come into our house. It would never happen and, even if it did, it wouldn't happen at our house.

[*The parent is trying to provide immediate security with factual information which they then reinforce with their own ability to protect their family.*]

Parent: I'm going to mention to your teacher that this game is causing you some problems and I think he will think that it isn't the right kind of game for children your age to play. Then tonight I'm going to show you all the things we have at our flat to keep us all really safe and I'm going to make sure that we know exactly who is coming to our house and when. Do you think that will help?

Depending on whether their response is yes or no, go with it, and ask if they think anything else will help. Then do the things you say you will do and check on it.

In all the above situations, the steps are pretty similar. The aim is to identify the fear or anxiety, show our child we are listening and are on their team and then show them that we are going to sort it out. But what do you do if your child doesn't know why they are scared?

Samir is a five-year-old who doesn't know why he has been feeling anxious. In Samir's case, we are going to put out an offering of possible options for our child's anxiety and see which they respond to.

Parent: I just wanted to chat for a few minutes about something I've been wondering about. I've noticed that for the past few weeks you have seemed a little worried / scared / stressed out / funny and I've been thinking about what might be going on.

Samir: I don't know why I'm feeling like this.

Parent: It must be hard to feel funny but not to know what's wrong. Maybe we can work it out together? How about I make some guesses and you see if any of them feel right?

[At this point, I would have my ideas prepared just in case. You want to have a few things you think might be right and a few things you are almost sure it isn't. Keep your face curious but positive. For a child who has recently started school and has had a new sibling, you might say:]

Parent: Is it maybe that going to your new school is different from nursery?

[Wait for a yes or a no.]

Parent: Is it maybe that the toys are not as good at this school as they were before? / Is it that the baby is sometimes with us when you just want it to be you and Daddy?

My experience has always shown that children will not say yes to something they don't mean, particularly if the conversation happens in a calm, quiet and connected way. You may also find that a child will say no but then come back to you later and say you were right.

In the conversation above, we are wondering about school anxiety and the anxiety brought on by displacement in a family. We will then work from what they say to find the details of the situation and to make a strategic plan.

These same principles apply whatever the age of your child. For a teenager whose parents have been through a recent divorce and is doing important exams, for example, you might say:

Parent: There are a lot of things going on for you at the moment. I know the last few months have been really difficult with Mum moving out and all the exam stress you're dealing with. Do you think it might be to do with either or both of them? Do you think something may be unresolved for you? Do you think there is anything I could do or say to help?

During this initial conversation, we are trying to set a fair, truthful and sensible tone to manage our child's reality. We will have an opportunity over time or in therapy to help our child manage the underlying feelings, fears or losses in the situation, but for now we are trying to show our child they are safe and their fears are being managed.

Brain-calming ideas

The first step to calming the brain is to show a child they are not alone by telling them you have noticed something is up and you are here with them as they go through it. We reinforce our ability to manage them by doing any of the below:

- Offering facts to match our safe worldview.
- Putting practical measures in place to help them.
- Monitoring and changing the plan as needed.
- Showing that we have the emotional capacity to hold whatever fear or worry comes up.
- Showing that we have the skill or can find someone with the skill to tackle the problem.
- Taking the worry onto ourselves and releasing our child by saying, 'Now I know about this, I'm in charge of it,' or 'Let me work out how we'll sort this out'.
- Showing our child that they can carry on in spite of this worry (but not expecting them to).
- Praising our child for their bravery and patience in managing this issue.

- Spending time with them not talking about this problem.
- Making time to manage this problem directly.
- Seeking additional support where needed.
- Being kind to them and ourselves as we navigate whatever is about to come along.
- Looking after ourselves so that our children can trust us to be OK for them or adding trustworthy support for our family for the times we cannot be available.

The process of calming children down works more easily if you are able to give them specific facts and information to reassure them, but this is not imperative.

Our aim is to listen to our child, see the fear their body has taken on and help them expel it and restore a feeling of safety.

Practical suggestions to help whatever the reason

Here are some practical ways you can help to reassure your child if they have become suddenly anxious.

Sound Off About Safety

If your child has been feeling generally anxious, showing how safe your home set-up is can make a huge difference. For example:

- **Do a home safety tour.** Explain: 'We have a big gate at the back of our house, we have a camera doorbell, I know exactly who is coming over to our house and I won't let anyone come over uninvited.'

- **Give facts about noises in the home.** 'That noise you heard in the night is most likely the heating coming on. Our heating is scheduled to come on at six so it starts powering up at five. Is that when you heard that noise?'

- **Talk about safety to your partner or other adults like a pilot.** Near your child but not to your child, call out: 'I'm locking the door for the night, honey, we aren't expecting any visitors. Will you check if the garden door is shut?' [Partner checks and locks back door.] 'Yes, sweetheart, all done for the night.'

  You don't have to use these nicknames if you use others! Do that for a month and see if your child seems noticeably calmer in the evening. This is more important if your child has experienced a real breach in safety like a burglary, watched something worrying on TV or seems jumpy and hypervigilant.

Talk About *Your* Skills

I find parents forget to say how good they are at things. We may think we aren't good at a lot or feel it would be boastful to say we are, but the upshot is we rarely tell our children how capable we are. Alternatively, I sometimes hear mums doing positive PR jobs for dads – 'Dad is so strong, he can fix anything' – but not for themselves. Proclaiming or discussing your skills can help children feel they can come to you and be supported if a problem arises. You may also explain, 'Yes, at our house, Daddy usually does the cooking but that's because he gets home earlier than I do. I can also cook and enjoy it but our schedule usually means he does.' It's good to show our children we can all do most things, which makes them feel that we can support them in any eventuality.

A Spoonful Not a Flood

Noted American psychiatrist Bruce Perry suggests using what he calls 'dosing'. Dosing is a method to keep a child inside their window of tolerance. The idea is that we dose against dysregulation by making small moments for distraction, connection and meeting your child's needs. For example, we may believe that we should rush through the process of getting our child up, dressed and off to school, but we may find that allowing for a more meandering route gets better results, as we move more calmly between moments and joke, dance or eat on the way out the door.

We may also believe that our child needs to talk deeply about their feelings to make progress, but under this model we can try peppering the serious conversations with moments of calm and fun in order to glean better results.

Add in More Family Fun

The part of our brain that controls emotions decides how we feel based on the chemical or neurotransmitter we are producing the most of at the time. Adding more fun, care-based or physical activities to our timetable can give relief from (cortisol-fuelled) anxiety in the short term by increasing the amount of serotonin, oxytocin, dopamine or endorphins in our child's brain. If you do it regularly, they will feel better and calmer more of the time.

Don't Be Afraid to Return to an Issue

If you have talked with your child and you think they may have kept something important to themselves, you've missed something or you could have handled the conversation better, go back in for another round. Set the right scene using the tips above and try again.

Find Someone Else to Help

Whether you need someone to rewire a plug and plaster the wall or pick your kids up on a Tuesday afternoon, ask for a favour from a neighbour or a friend or hire someone – but know that you can't and don't have to do everything yourself. Support for an anxious child or a stressed-out parent comes in many forms.

Manage Your Own Self-care and Relationship Vibe

Hypervigilant and anxious children will have a super-sensitive barometer for how happy and safe a family home is.

They will see angry looks and hear your tone. Make time to fill your own cup as well as working on your relationship with your partner to try to improve the feeling of a visible and positive relationship.

Try to focus on keeping inside your window of tolerance by allowing both you and your partner to take breaks and calm down if you get angry with each other.

Make Loving Time Together a Priority

Are you a cuddly family? Do you tell your child how much you like and love them? Are there practical ways you could show your child you think they are great just as they are? Say it! Sing it! Write it! Find a way you feel comfortable with to show your child how special you think they are. Sit next to each other and enjoy it.

I regularly recommend that families look at their week and the way they are constantly rushing between scouts and gymnastics, chess club and the sea cadets, piano and football practice, etc., and think how many minutes they all get to be together as a family. Many of us are trying to feed our relationships with our families in snatched moments between activities our children will only do for a short time. Think about this one question: when they grow up, will you and your child wish you'd had more rushed afternoons where they'd choked down a sandwich outside the village hall as they pulled on their shin pads, or will you wish you had made more time to be together in the week? Is there one activity or one evening you could clear to make time with your family without having to rush?

Body-calming ideas

Our body may need time to catch up to our mind when anxiety and its chemical components are present. A hypervigilant body takes time to calm down and understand the threat is no longer present. We can help this process by consistently showing the body it is safe and has enough time to relax and recharge.

This is easier done than said – here are some practical ways to do it:

Shut the Door

Something as simple as shutting the door to the room your child is in so they don't have to keep checking for variables can give our kids and their bodies some needed rest after a day of hypervigilance. This way they know that whatever is happening in the room will stay the same until someone opens the door again.

Spend Time With Animals

If you have pets or know someone who does, get your children as close as you can safely. Animals centre the body and give us immediate access to oxytocin, serotonin and dopamine, particularly if we get to touch and play with them. Perhaps try visiting a city farm or petting zoo?

Spend Time Outside

Taking children outside to a park or green space is always beneficial, whether you are going for a calm walk in nature or burning off extra energy with some physical activity. Either way, it should lead to better sleep.

Firework idea

Did you know that seeing six trees is enough to change our eyes from hard fascination (the kind of intense focus our eyes do on a laptop or phone) to soft fascination – a relaxation of the eye that lets us take in more light, widen the view we are seeing and relax our bodies by telling us that we have officially stopped working and are allowed some respite?

Do Things to Trigger Your Body's Other Chemicals

Exercise, being with friends, playing games, ticking some items off your to-do list. Find a way to give the cortisol a break and do something to add some positive chemicals into your system.

Try Yoga and Mindfulness

Still activities that cause us to slow down and breathe more deeply can make a huge difference to our anxiety. This is because allowing yourself to sit still and breathe is the opposite to what you would do if you were being chased by a predator. When we make our body still by choice, our body thinks that we are safe.

Improve Your Sleep

Prioritising everyone's sleep can make a huge difference to the levels of cortisol we will feel the next day. If possible, get yourself and your child to bed earlier or make modifications for better sleep, like increasing the darkness and temperature in the bedroom.

Make Time for Imaginative Play, Storytelling and Creating Art

You can be sure that if you were in danger, you wouldn't be whipping out your easel and brushes. Making time for still, positive and creative activities tells the brain we are safe and can settle and enjoy different chemicals and experiences. Make sure the activities you are setting up don't make you even more stressed by limiting the materials and the location so you can relax while they create.

Connect Physically

Oxytocin is produced by hand-holding, cuddling and stroking – but high fives, sitting next to someone and even smiling also increase the connective chemicals between us. If your kids are walking somewhere, aim to hold their hand. If they are watching TV, sit next to them.

> **Firework idea**
>
> **Think of a funny, easy-to-remember secret handshake and add it in to your goodbye routine.**

Be Reliable

Our kids' bodies will calm down when they feel they mostly know what is going on. Being reliable or making sure the schedule your children are running on is reliable can make a huge difference. If your child usually goes somewhere or is picked up by someone, make it reliable, and if there is going to be a change, let them know. You are only as reliable as the information you give.

Add a Feeling of Relaxation to Your Child's Timetable

Look at your child's schedule. How many days do they stay out of the house after school? Is there extended time together at the weekend?

Firework idea

Tell your child that as soon as you get home for the evening or the weekend, you will all relax. Your home is there to let the fear switch off and the body relax. Maybe light a candle and have a cuddle on the sofa. Aim to make your home the safest, calmest place your kids ever go!

The need for care and connection

If your child believes in their relationship with you and the way you care for them, that can be enough to fight off worries. Having a reliable, loving and sensible parent on their team who fights for their needs, listens and acts with kindness and is capable enough that they trust you to manage them, even in extremis, is the key to helping children.

How to do it:

- Be seen.
- Be present.
- Be kind.
- Be reliable.
- Be loving.

For my little client Max with the Zorro teachers, even though he had been worried for a while, he was feeling much better and happy at school once we showed him the pictures his teachers had of them dressed up in their costumes with no masks. They explained to him it had been them and they thought the children knew and would find it funny. They were sorry they hadn't considered this possible fear and it has been taken out of planning for future year groups. They took him on a safety tour of the school and mostly kept the classroom door shut for the rest of the term. At home, his parents worked on calming his body with quieter after-school evenings, outdoor play and 'co-pilot talking' about how capable they were and how safe the house was.

And that was it. That was enough to silence the fear, reduce the cortisol and get that little boy back to school with a big smile on his face.

Books to help your suddenly anxious child		
Children	Teens	Adults
My Monster and Me by Nadiya Hussain	Don't Worry, Be Happy by Poppy O'Neill	The Opposite of Worry: The Playful Parenting Approach to Childhood Anxieties and Fears by Lawrence J. Cohen
The Worrysaurus by Rachel Bright	What to Do When You Worry Too Much by Dawn Heubner	
Ruby's Worry by Tom Percival		Under Pressure: Confronting the Epidemic of Stress and Anxiety in Girls by Lisa Damour
The Huge Bag of Worries by Virginia Ironside	A Smart Girl's Guide: Worry by Nancy Holyoke	
Find Your Calm by Gabi Garcia	Unstuck by Barbara Dee	

Four

Help! My Child Has Always Been Anxious

One in five children are born highly sensitive and con-sequently struggle in some way with routine things most people take for granted. Highly sensitive children seem to process and react to their environment more acutely than other children and can struggle socially, at school, with rela-tionships or even with daily events like eating, sleeping or leaving home.

Why are some children more likely to be highly sensitive?

- **Genetics** play a huge part in how sensitive a child will be. Inherited sensitivity, genetically inherited conditions or neurodivergence can be part of the reason some children find the world overwhelming or wrestle with society's expectations.

- Conversely, a child's **natural personality** can be very dif-ferent from their parents' and the rest of a family's. Each child is an individual. Although the atmosphere in the wider family is influential, this child's reaction to events is strictly their own.

- **Environmental factors** can play a part in a child's devel-opment. Stress or trauma for the biological mother, drug or alcohol use during pregnancy, birth trauma or early attachment problems could impair a child's resilience to experiences.

- **Neurological and health differences** such as autism spectrum disorder (ASD), attention deficit hyperactivity disorder (ADHD), sensory processing issues, blindness, deafness, speech difficulties, chronic illness and many other conditions can contribute to a child's list of dys-regulating factors. Anxiety is a common comorbidity/ additional diagnosis or symptom that comes with every kind of neurodivergence. A recent survey by the National Autistic Society found that 47 per cent of autistic people are considered to have severe anxiety. A similar estimate of 50 per cent of those with ADHD suffer from anx-iety. Those with learning difficulties such as dyslexia, dyspraxia, dyscalculia, dysgraphia or a sensory process-ing condition that inhibits learning will no doubt find school and other situations needing focus or processing extremely anxiety-inducing.
- **Parenting style** can affect a child's ability to manage in the world or cause them to feel fearful. Parents use their rules, structures and personalities to prepare, arm and translate the world for their children.
- **Cultural and social influences** may make a child who would blend comfortably into one family stand out uncomfortably in another. A shy child in an outgoing family or a timid child in an adventurous family will seem more anxious in comparison with everyone else. A dyslexic child may stand out more in a family of high

academic achievers. In some cultures, a sensitive boy may be viewed much more critically than a sensitive girl.

Firework idea

When talking about your children, do not label them: instead use positive language. Aim to use a word you would be happy if someone said about you. Think of the difference between 'takes her ideas seriously' versus 'stubborn'; 'takes his time' versus 'lazy'; 'aware of her feelings' versus 'sensitive'.

How do you know if you have a highly sensitive/ anxious child?

- Your child has acute sensitivity to sensory stimulus – loud noises, hot or cold weather, smells, bright lights or the feeling of a certain material against their skin.
- Your child is deeply affected by things they watch and hear. Your child may have low tolerance for scary things or situations of jeopardy.
- Your child has very specific food preferences.
- Your child struggles to sleep calmly through the night.
- Your child overthinks other people's behaviour or has a tendency to be left out or feel left out.
- Your child may know what is going on in your home or your world without needing to be told. They may surprise you with questions about things you are sure they couldn't know.

- They have strong emotional reactions to any issue or problem.
- They feel very offended and emotionally wounded when they hurt themselves, even superficially.
- They have a vivid imagination and are naturally creative.
- They can take criticism or correction very personally and let it break down their self-esteem quickly.
- They can become easily overstimulated, quickly overexcited, angry or upset and find it hard to calm down.
- They may need quiet time or to spend time alone.
- They have the capacity to learn to a high level and can understand concepts and subtleties beyond their years.

The revolutionary book by Dr W. Thomas Boyce, *The Orchid and the Dandelion*, highlights the theory that sensitive children are born with biological differences to other children. Just as orchids need more tending than other flowers, sensitive children require more nurturing than others in order to thrive. If you carefully nurture an orchid child, they will always grow into somebody special, interesting and beautiful.

As anxiety comes from feeling unsafe and our body's primary directive is to keep us alive, children who are naturally sensitive or have neurodivergence or disability are more likely to feel they are at risk. It makes sense that they are naturally more susceptible to anxiety, fear and panic.

Our job is to give our little orchid babies a safe haven that is tailor-made for them. This will help them gain the skills they need to manage what seem to them potentially worrying experiences.

Let's start by building resilience

Sensitive children may seem to lack resilience, but how about looking at their behaviour differently? After all, sensitive children show remarkable resilience every day just by waking up each morning and functioning in a world that scares and overwhelms them. Our role is to quieten the noise, reassure them, explain the parts of daily life that feel overwhelming and provide consistent, visible support.

Our aim is to teach them effective methods to manage their needs, emotions and relationships and we can achieve this by using some or all of the techniques and lifestyle choices below.

Teaching independent skills

According to a 75-year-long Harvard University study, children who do chores at home are likely to be more successful in life than those who don't. This is because not only does performing helpful tasks teach responsibility, it also makes children feel like valued members of a team contributing towards a common goal.

For highly sensitive children, make an age-appropriate chore list. Focus on tasks they can achieve on their own. Making them feel capable will have a considerable impact on their self-esteem, staving off the worrying feeling they cannot manage for even a short time by themselves.

Showing children they can meet their most important needs can help them feel self-sufficient, which significantly decreases anxiety. The child knows they can manage most things competently and is likely to absorb more complicated skills as they grow older. See if your child can do any/all of the following: organise their own breakfast or packed lunch, brush their hair or teeth, wash their face, hands and hair, understanding directions, keep their possessions in order, dress themselves appropriately for hot and cold weather, start a conversation with someone or ask for something they need independently.

Supporting growth mindset – no one is brilliant at everything straight away

Fostering a 'growth mindset' is essential for all children, but it's particularly important for highly sensitive children. This is the idea that no one is good at something straight away and that anything worth doing will require practice. We have capacity to improve if we work hard and ask for help. Growth mindset encourages failure as a step on the way to mastery. It shows us no one is perfect at anything without practice and work, we are not in competition with anyone else and, even if we are not especially gifted at something, if we stick at it, we will do it more effectively tomorrow.

A supporting growth mindset helps children not to despair. Today may be tough. Tomorrow will be a little better. This helps highly sensitive children feel that parameters are moveable and we can improve and change. Being a family that promotes a growth mindset will build resilience and help our children understand we believe in hard work, tenacity and trying our very best to get the results we want.

Here are some tips to help your child understand the concept of growth mindset:

- Focus on adding the word 'yet'. When your child says, 'I can't do it', add the word 'yet' and remind them that all important skills require practice.
- Share stories of times when you couldn't do something but managed it in the end. Make sure the story is age-appropriate and not worrying for your child.
- Praise hard work and creativity over winning or perfect outcomes.
- When praising or correcting your child's behaviour make clear what you appreciated or did not like. Be specific. Change 'Well done!' for 'I loved the effort you put into your picture', or 'You were such a kind teammate today. You really looked out for the others.' Instead of 'Stop that!', try: 'When you use your hands to hurt people, I will have to stop you.' Or: 'I saw how you asked your brother and then didn't listen to what he said. We have to let others decide what they want to do.'

Firework idea

Try one new thing with your child every day. Reward them for taking part. Ask them to identify what they think they did well.

Provide clear timetables and plans

Having clear information about what they are going to do or where they are going can help highly sensitive children feel calmer.

- Have a visible timetable of the week in your home that your child can check (or be reminded to check). Colour in their favourite things in a different colour so they can see there are very few days or even hours to wait between the things they love.
- Organise stations in your home to help your child be sure they have all they need: shoes, school bag, PE kit. You may need to provide visual checklists, boxes that always house the same thing and hooks that are the right size for a small person to reach.
- Be a communicative personal assistant. When information or plans change, let your hypersensitive child know. Call the school office, change the family planner or send a text. Help your child feel they know who is visiting and give them time to prepare for the new plan.

Firework idea

If your child thrives with a clear timetable, make one for holiday time too. It can be much looser than a school schedule and have vaguer outlines like 'free play' or 'crafts or building'. Add any special events too. This will help a child feel that they can get through the tricky transition to holidays while still feeling held and looked after.

Practise gratitude

Helping highly sensitive children practise gratitude can help them see their world in a positive light. A 2008 study by Algoe, Haidt and Gable found that gratitude boosts positive emotions and leads to greater overall wellbeing by enhancing positive social interactions and relationships. Research has shown that gratitude helps build resilience by focusing on the positive aspects of life, which buffers against stress and negative emotions.

By helping our children to regularly notice and discuss the good things in their life, the more they will spot the good in the world. It can help them to become a more 'glass-half-full' kind of person, which will help them in tougher times.

Ask your child every few days: 'What were you grateful for today?' Help them practise spotting the good, great and special in every day. They can write their thoughts down in a gratitude journal so you can look back at their most positive moments at a later date.

Teach kids to HALT

Our highly sensitive children may be prone to getting overwhelmed during transitions or when they have to make a decision. It's important to help them realise they need to HALT and sort out their needs. HALT stands for:

- H: Hungry
- A: Angry
- L: Lonely
- T: Tired

Using this to identify the feeling underneath the anxiety makes it much more manageable to the child, as it means they can fix any of those problems simply by eating, finding someone to help them calm down or feel included, or resting. For neurodivergent children, a simple body check-in like this can make all the difference to managing a social or educational issue.

If your child is getting upset, you can say, 'HALT, let's see what your body is feeling. Ask your body if it's hungry.' Go through each one until your child says what is bothering them and then show them how they can manage it.

- H: Have snacks in their bag if they are regularly overwhelmed because they are hungry.

- A: Practise calm breathing and show them how they can use their body physically but in a safe way to get the anger out.
- L: Help them learn how to ask another child to play or ask an adult for support.
- T: Teach them it's safe and we're allowed to rest when our body tells us to.

Firework idea

If your child is upset and breathing exercises are too much for them, talk about things in the present – the colour of your T-shirt, whether the window is usually open or shut, whether it was faster or slower to come in the car today than walking yesterday. This allows a child to engage the thinking brain in the prefrontal cortex, moving the focus away from the reptilian brain that controls the flight or fight response. It grounds them and brings them back to the here and now.

Teach the catastrophe scale

Try teaching your kids this useful scale to help them understand the different levels of danger:

5: EMERGENCY – Someone is hurt or in danger; you will need help from an adult, maybe the police, the fire brigade or an ambulance. Perhaps there has been a fire, you have witnessed a crime or someone has hurt themselves badly. Reassure your anxious child it is very, very rare to have this kind of emergency, but knowing the difference is important.

4: BIG PROBLEM – You have a problem that you can't fix without help but the other person wouldn't need to be from emergency services. For example, you are lost, someone is being unkind to you, you need help to calm down or someone has hurt themselves and needs first aid.

3: MEDIUM PROBLEM – This is something you can manage if someone would help you, such as being hungry, feeling sick or scared, the feeling that someone or something is bothering you.

2: LITTLE PROBLEM – This is a problem that would be fixed faster or more effectively with help. You spilled something, you can't reach something, you need someone to open a packet. You could struggle with it but a little help would go a long way to what you need.

1: GLITCH – A glitch is a little problem that you can fix yourself. You need a red pencil and don't have one at your table, but you know where to get one. You aren't sure if there is someone in the loo, so you push the door to see if it's locked.

Once your child has learned the scale, when they have a problem, you can say, 'What kind of problem is it? What help do you think you might need?'

The more you use it in your home the more your kids will say, 'No need, it's just a glitch.'

Using proprioception to calm our children's bodies

Your proprioceptive sense is your ability to know where your body is in space. As adults, we have years of experience honing this skill. If I asked you to shut your eyes and walk to the other side of the room, you will probably have an instinct about how far away it is and you would be unlikely to smash into the wall. Having this skill calms the body as it helps it know we would be able to safely make and execute an escape route in a dangerous situation. Children with an underdeveloped proprioceptive sense can experience greater anxiety as they can't use the information to calm the mind.

Studies in the past twenty years, such as those by Miller et al. (2007) and Schaaf and Nightlinger (2007), found proprioceptive activities contribute to better emotional regulation and reduce anxiety levels in children. They also highlighted that this type of activity, as part of a sensory diet, helps to improve the self-regulation and adaptive behaviours of children with autism spectrum disorder (ASD). (A sensory diet is a plan we can put in place for highly sensitive/neurodivergent children that considers their sensory input both at home and elsewhere, for example giving the child the option to wear headphones if the noise of assembly is too much.)

Different children will respond well to different kinds of

proprioceptive inputs or experiences. Try to recall if your child likes to swing, squash or crash, or what they enjoy doing in a park. You can recreate this at home to bring a sense of calmness to the body.

There are eight different kinds of proprioceptive activities. Once you have identified your child's favourites, you can vary the ways they engage with them to keep them exciting and fit them into your schedule. These kinds of activities aid proprioception as they engage the ears and eyes, which then send signals down the vagus nerve (the nerve that meanders down from our face to our gut) that tell us we can relax as we know where we are and we're in control. Try to add at least one of these activities on most days:

- **Deep-pressure activities:** Massages, giving big tight hugs, using weighted blankets or stuffed animals, using very tight bed sheets at night, squeezing playdough or doing a music-based workout with dough (search 'dough disco'), using stress balls or squeezy fidget toys, rolling your child up in a blanket tightly like a burrito, squashing them between pillows and pretending they are a sandwich.
- **Movement-based activities:** Playing hopscotch or jumping over obstacles, dancing to music with various intensity levels, using a skipping rope or jumping over a rope held close to the ground, rolling down hills or slopes, using scooter boards for pushing and pulling activities, jumping on a trampoline, jumping jacks, using a swing or rolling over a therapy ball.

- **Coordination and balance activities:** Sitting and bouncing on exercise balls, using balance boards or wobble boards, walking on a taped line or balance beam, practising standing on one foot or doing the yoga tree pose, using space hoppers or bouncing balls, creating obstacle courses that require crawling, jumping, balancing and climbing, riding a bike or scooter to develop balance and coordination.
- **Resistance activities:** Using TheraBands or exercise bands for resistance exercises, putting them on the front two legs of your child's chair to give their feet a feeling of resistance, playing tug-of-war with a rope or resistance band, pushing against walls or heavy furniture in a controlled manner, using rope ladders or nets for climbing activities, rolling large balls of dough or playdough, making bread or pizza.
- **Joint compression and stretching:** Hanging from monkey bars or pull-up bars, playing games on a soft surface, getting gently squished by pillows, stretching and pulling resistance bands in different directions, doing planks, push-ups or wall push-ups, walking like different animals (e.g. bear walks, crab walks, frog jumps) to engage various muscles and joints.
- **Fine motor proprioceptive activities:** Threading beads or uncooked penne, cutting through different materials, such as playdough, foam, cardboard or paper, using tools like a hole punch or stapler, playing with clothes pegs, squishy toys or stress balls.
- **Heavy work activities:** Creating an obstacle course where your children have to move heavy objects from one place

to another, getting children working in the garden (e.g. digging, raking and pushing a wheelbarrow filled with soil or plants), getting them to help out with bigger household tasks like vacuuming or mopping floors. Find good reasons for your child to carry heavy things like helping with grocery bags, laundry baskets or moving small pieces of furniture.

- **Oral proprioceptive activities:** Eating chewy or crunchy foods like dried fruit, sugar-free gum or raw vegetables, blowing bubbles, blowing up balloons, blowing through a straw, using chewy tubes, specially designed chewing necklaces or oral motor tools designed for sensory input, drinking thick liquids like smoothies through a straw, using vibrating oral tools for input to the jaw and mouth, playing with whistles or kazoos, blowing through small wind instruments.

Sleep hygiene

Helping sensitive, anxious children start the day with the most energy and focus will only be achievable if your child is getting as much good-quality sleep as possible. Although anxiety and neurodivergence can affect sleep in lots of negative ways, we can improve our child's 'sleep hygiene' by adopting practices and habits that promote a better night's rest. Here are some strategies to enhance sleep hygiene:

- Look at the school week as a climb uphill from Monday to Friday. For children masking fears or neurological difference, it can be exhausting to hold in thoughts, misunderstandings and perceived negative behaviour or actions all week. Consider that some children will need the evenings after school from Wednesday to Friday to be less strenuous. Aim for fewer after-school activities later in the week, easy-to-cook-and-clean family dinners to speed the evening routine up, and consider that from the moment they get home, they should have the feeling they are on a smooth, calm slide to bedtime (preferably a little earlier than normal). Bath them early, get them in their pyjamas and make the evening feel easy and positive.

Firework idea

On a day when your child is really struggling and it feels like all is lost, ask, 'What can we do to save the day?' Give manageable options and allow your child the freedom to pick. Use this idea in reverse too: on days where your child had a tough moment and got out of it, ask, 'What did you do to save today?' Use their own tips for other days.

- Limit exposure to screens. There is more and more data to suggest that children are affected by blue light and that it delays natural production of melatonin and the feeling of sleepiness in children. Understand that video games, videos of people playing video games and media consumed alone on small screens can lead to increased agitation and dysregulation. Even watching on a larger screen as a team in one place is more calming for the body and will increase oxytocin before bed. Aim to turn off all tech for children at least an hour before they go to sleep. Look at the guidelines for screen time from the World Health Organization to see if your children are using screens too frequently.

- Try to give children chances to talk about their worries or problems earlier in the day so that they aren't full up with them just as they are about to be alone in the dark with their thoughts.

- During term time in particular, try to put kids to bed at a similar time each night, about twelve hours after they woke up for primary-school-aged children and about fourteen hours after wake-up for children over thirteen. Keeping to a simple sleep schedule tells our children's bodies when to expect to be tired and helps them sleep better.

- Aim to make bedtimes feel full of love, relaxation and a bit of fun. We can help anxious children sail into sleep by having a predictable routine and by adding in moments for laughter. This connection will help them fill up with positive chemicals before they get into bed to counteract their natural anxiety.

- Try to set your child's room up for the best sleep possible by making it dark, cool and quiet.

- Help your child to associate their bed with sleep by doing other activities out of the room or not on the bed.

- Expose your child to natural light by opening the curtains as early as possible after waking up and get outside during the day too.

Firework idea

Consider that by Thursday each week, your highly sensitive child has survived mostly without your protection in the real world and is likely to be exhausted from masking or trying as hard as they can to complete tasks. So why not make Thursday or Friday evening into a spa night? Play some calming music, give them a foot massage and put some bubbles in a lovely warm bath. Show your child they are allowed to relax and recharge.

Other possible interventions:

- **Mindfulness:** Teaching children mindfulness skills can be very helpful: they will learn that we do not have to listen to all our thoughts and can find calm, even in a busy world with a busy brain. Look for a local children's mindfulness group or practitioner, watch children's mindfulness videos on YouTube and sit with your child to help anchor them and keep them going.

- **Emotional Freedom Technique (EFT):** Often just called tapping, this is a method of teaching mindfulness where you do not have to be still or quiet. This works well for children with ADHD and those who need to be busy to be calm. Look up videos online, or order the book *Gorilla Thumps and Bear Hugs* by Alex Ortner to explain EFT to younger children. You can also find practitioners who can teach your child EFT in person or online.

- **Yoga:** Yoga can help children find a sense of power in stillness and develop strength. It is an easy proprioceptive activity you can do at home or in a class. You can watch yoga videos like Cosmic Kids Yoga on YouTube, you can buy Yoga Pretzels children's yoga cards and I recommend *Good Night Yoga* by Mariam Gates for a book to read at bedtime with children under ten to add a few calming moves to your night-time routine.

- **Handwriting support:** Children with lots of worries often struggle at school. Having handwriting coaching for a short block of time can help take something off our child's mind if it helps them master this skill. You can also teach your child to type to help support their written communication. I recommend Dance Mat Typing which is free on the BBC website.

- **Art:** Art classes, particularly those that use clay, can help children receive sensory input, give opportunities to find other talents, express themselves and find a sense of calm in exploration and creation. Google local art or pottery classes, short photography courses for teenagers, or ask a school art teacher for things you could do at home. Watch drawing videos together to help them increase their drawing skills over time and add to the things they feel positive about in their armoury of talents.

- **Martial arts:** All martial arts have the ability to help children feel a sense of control and mastery of their body. Helping anxious children understand how strong and powerful they can be can make a huge difference in how permeable they feel and whether they know they can manage in any situation.

- **Occupational therapy:** This can be extremely helpful for anxious children as it can help to explain whether a child is sensitive for an emotional, sensory or physical reason. The occupational therapist will help children identify triggers in the environment and learn skills to feel more in control of their bodies, such as balancing and having the same control over different sides of the body. There is increasing evidence in the OT community that some anxiety and developmental issues come from children retaining reflexes similar to the startle reflex or finger gripping we see in babies, so helping children to reduce these early reflexes can aid their development and help them interact and concentrate better.

- **Cranial osteopathy:** This can help to soothe children's bodies, resulting in deeper breathing and a feeling of calmness. It can reduce inflammation and increase their sense of control over time.

Books to help your always anxious child		
Children	**Teens**	**Adults**
Anxious Ninja by Mary Nhin *Help Your Dragon Deal with Anxiety* by Steve Herman *When Things Get Too Loud: A Story About Sensory Overload* by Anne Alcott	*No Worries! An Activity Book for Children Who Sometimes Feel Anxious or Stressed* by Dr Sharie Coombes *A Little Spot of Anxiety: A Story About Calming Your Worries* by Diane Alber	*The Whole-Brain Child: 12 Revolutionary Strategies to Nurture Your Child's Developing Mind* by Daniel J. Siegel and Tina Payne Bryson

How Big Are Your Worries Little Bear? by Jayneen Sanders *Too Much!: An Overwhelming Day* by Jolene Gutiérrez	*Hey Warrior* by Karen Young *Outsmarting Worry: An Older Kid's Guide to Managing Anxiety* by Dawn Huebner	*The Orchid and the Dandelion: Why Sensitive People Struggle and How All Can Thrive* by W. Thomas Boyce

Five

Help! My Child's Separation Anxiety is Giving Me Anxiety!

What are the very real fears hiding behind this anxiety?

- The fear you could be left alone.
- The fear your parent will never come back.
- The fear you will not be looked after.
- The fear the adults looking after you will not manage your needs in the way your parents might.
- The fear no one will help you.

Elia had settled well at his new nursery school. After ten days of transition, just as his keyworker predicted, he had found his happy place. He loved it! He came home covered in sand and paint and sang all the upbeat songs he had learned there as he played at home. The year was passing by at speed, one happy day after another, when, seemingly out of nowhere, Elia began to show acute separation anxiety. He would scream and cry from the moment he woke up to the moment he reached the school doors. He would kick and scratch his parents as they put his nursery uniform on and kick his shoes off. He would climb his parents like trees at the door to the classroom and cling on like a monkey.

I received a frantic email asking if they should immediately change nurseries or if his mum should quit her job and start home-schooling him. They were scared any number of horrific things could have happened to him. We booked in an assessment session and I got to work.

I sat down with Elia and asked him about school and home. He could easily list the things and people he loved at both. We talked about his routine, how he would get to school, who picked him up, what he would wear. I checked for sensory issues – was it a loud classroom? A tight uniform? I checked for social issues – were there naughty children in his class? 'Hurty' children? Shouty children? I asked about the stories they had read and the toys they played with in the nursery. NOTHING. Then I asked about his mum. I said, 'What does Mummy do when you are at school?'

'She teaches big children!' he said. Mum was a university lecturer. She had organised her schedule so she could pick him up four days a week.

Mum had taught him a little sing-song phrase: 'On Monday, Tuesday, Wednesday, Thursday, Mummy will always come.' Elia happily repeated it to me.

I said, 'And that always happens?'

'Umm . . . umm.' He started to cry.

His mum explained that about five weeks before, she had had a sick bug. She had not been able to pick him up as she had been doubled over on the floor. Instead, his grandma had picked him up on time and taken him straight home. It seemed the shock of not seeing his mum at the gate then spotting her lying on the floor in the bathroom on his return home had destroyed his sense of security. This was a one-off event, carefully managed by his closest adults to have the least possible impact on him, yet it had been enough to instil profound separation anxiety in this normally happy boy.

We often find that although any change in a parent's behaviour has a massive effect on children, the absence of the primary caregiver shocks children to the core. Why are they so dramatically derailed? The answer is crystal clear: when the primary caregiver is not where he or she is supposed to be, they feel profound fear because they know if they are not looked after or their needs are not met, they could die.

I explained the impact of this information and we immediately changed Elia's mum's phrase to: 'On Monday, Tuesday, Wednesday, Thursday, Mummy will always come' – and then they would whisper, 'Unless she's got a really good reason not to, in which case she will send Grandma or someone else you know and love!'

I sent Mum for a check-up at the GP so she could tell Elia in good faith that she was well and didn't think there would be any reason she would be ill again.

Mum told Elia that if there were any changes, she would call the nursery school and let them know. Only a few weeks later, once he had returned more calmly to school, a big test came up. Mum's work schedule had changed and she would miss one pick-up.

She told him in the morning who was coming, she loudly told his teacher too and she even called one more time near the end of the day to make sure Elia remembered.

The preparation and direct attack on the primal fear that 'Mummy wasn't OK' and wouldn't be able to care for him was immediately pushed away by having a safe plan that showed she was thinking about him and looking after him even if she wasn't there. She did this by setting up special activities for him at home on those days, having his favourite snacks picked out for him in the morning and calling him to say she was on the way home. He didn't need to question her ability to care for him even for a second. He was calm again.

Firework idea

Focus on 'mind-mindedness' – the feeling of holding someone in mind even when you are not together. This is an extremely powerful tool for children. Bringing something home for them or telling them something you heard in the day that they would be interested in makes a child feel cared for even when you aren't around.

Let's talk about separation anxiety

Separation anxiety is an extremely normal part of a child's development. Every child will go through at least one phase in their first six years of life.

The most common stages are:

- At around six or seven months old, babies become more aware of their surroundings and begin to develop object permanence, which means they start to understand that an object, place or person continues to exist even when you can't see it. As this starts to develop, children begin to notice when their parents leave the room and it makes them panicky and confused. They are still getting to grips with object permanence; the concept isn't yet embedded in their minds so they can't be sure you are coming back.
- Between ten and eighteen months, separation anxiety increases. It can pop up at any time until children are three years old. It happens because as children get older, they have more awareness of where everything and everyone is and how the family systems work, so when they change, that feels chaotic and worrying.
- When children start going to school or nursery, it is common to see separation anxiety. It makes sense. It is the first major period of separation from a parent that children will face. This is coupled with the

obvious contrast between school and home. School is a bigger, louder place with a large group of unknown adults and children. Adjusting can take a while.

- Separation anxiety can also occur at the start of more formal schooling as children comprehend they will always be separated at least part of the time from their parents and the situation will continue for the foreseeable future.

- We may also see separation anxiety at any age when there is change or difficulty in a child's home life. Divorce, moving house, family illness and many other events make children reluctant to be separated from their parents or afraid to leave their home in case something bad or sad happens.

Firework idea

Always tell your child if you are leaving; let them know early if they will be asleep when you leave. Setting the tone that you will leave and then come back in a reliable way helps separation and relationship connection forever. Your child must trust you to leave and then return. When we don't tell them, they can be constantly on edge, thinking we might leave at any time, which leads to greater separation anxiety.

How do we help children with separation anxiety?

I would like you to hold two things in mind as we manage separation anxiety.

1. Separation anxiety is extremely normal and should stop relatively quickly. So, we can stay calm as we know this should be over soon.
2. This doesn't mean we can't put in extra support to speed the process and help at each stage.

Here are some practical ideas to help your child cope with being separated from you:

For Children Under One Year

- Organise your days in a reliable way. A 2014 study found that babies as young as a few months can recognise and are calmed by predictable routines.
- Aim to make your goodbye clear but short. If you have to leave, tell your baby and then go. Any additional back and forth can add stress and confusion.
- Practise short separations – you can even make up reasons to leave the house for a few minutes. These will help to confirm that you will return each time. Your child will build up a base of experiences they can draw on as their object permanence improves.
- Aim to stay calm. It can be very upsetting for parents when they have to leave a distressed baby, but remember that you trust the person you have left the baby with.

Now you must trust them to look after the baby as you leave. Ask them to message you as soon as the baby has calmed down. Focus on what you have to do and breathe deeply as you try to wait for the message. Looking fearful or upset can cause the baby to feel mistrust and fear too.

- Consider using the same toy, music, blanket or baby sling to give comfort and a sense of routine at the moment when the baby is being left.
- Engage in bonding activities with your baby: cuddling, singing, reading, playing. Give your baby a feeling of calm connection when you are at home with them.
- Aim to only leave your baby with people they have met before.

If your child goes to childcare:

- Share your routines and comfort objects.
- Encourage the relationship your child has with their key workers.
- Make time to introduce them to the setting and the adults there slowly.
- Ask them to be positive but honest with you about how your baby is doing in their care.
- Ask them to engage in comforting activities and make time to hold and rock your baby.

It is important to remember you will manage this change better too if you are prioritising your mental health and, if possible, your sleep.

Firework idea

Add peekaboo and hide and seek into your repertoire of activities at any age. This allows children to practise separation and reuniting in a safe and fun way.

For Toddlers

- Start by creating a goodbye ritual: a phrase, handshake, big cuddle. Aim to connect and have a laugh and do it every day.
- Keep goodbyes quick.
- Practise shorter separations before longer ones like a nursery day.
- Keep a smile on your face. We can make our children feel our nerves, making them believe they can't trust the people they are left with, if our facial expression implies we are unhappy leaving them.
- Do a 'talk through' about what to expect in the day, for example what fun things they could do at school. Also tell them some of the nice things you are going to do while you are away and then tell them when you will be back.
- Find a simple way to explain the routine of your week to your child. Consider having a visual timetable that shows which days they go to nursery and who will take and collect them. Explain there may be changes, but you will always try to let them know.
- Help your child practise skills they may need when you aren't there: putting their coat on, going to the loo, asking

for food or drink. If your child is too little to talk, practise tapping and pointing at the things they want.

- If you have gone out, you could call and check in but this may also interrupt your child's flow. You could send a video message for the adult in charge to play at a point where they think it will fit better into the events of the day.
- Let your child know that you understand it is hard, and that you love them and will miss them while you are out. Explain that you know the adult in charge is very clever, sensible and fun and they have all they need to look after them.

Firework idea

Find something to connect you when you are not together. Colour a heart on your hand and do the same on theirs, spray a bit of your perfume onto their school jumper, give them your business card or a copy of a photo to keep in their pocket. Try not to choose anything that would cause a problem if they lose it!

For Children Starting Nursery or School

- From the time you accept your place or have a start date, start your positive PR campaign for the school, the adults, the toys, the children. If there is something good you could say, say it! You are promoting positivity and safety and telling anyone who wants to listen. Say things like, 'Hey Auntie, did you know at Millie's new school all the adults are so kind and nice, they have a big playground and they have a special lady who helps when you hurt yourself. Isn't that so cool?!'

- Get skilled up! Parents learn to understand their children's communication and often pre-empt what children are about to say – but their school or nursery carers won't have that knowledge. Helping children feel comfortable in a new place starts with giving them the tools to get what they need. Help them prepare by getting them to practise asking for things clearly.

- Help them listen to their body and ask for water, food, the loo, a cuddle, or help to reach something. If they have delayed speech, show them to touch the teacher's arm for attention and point at what they need.

- Give context. Before your start date, show your child where school is. Practise your walk to school, talk about the children, adults and objects they will encounter there. If possible, meet up with other families and children who will attend. If you have a school tour or a stay-and-play before you start, take photos and show them to your child over the summer when you talk about school.

Firework idea

Walk or drive past the school a few times before you attend and tell your child to point and shout, 'That's my school!' This begins a positive association and connection before they even arrive.

- Set up clear routines. Children thrive when they know what will happen next. Try to explain the day in the same words. Use 'first', 'next' and 'last' to explain what will happen and in what order.
- Focus on sleep.
- Minimise stress.
- Give a sense of ownership with uniform and bookbag.
- Consider healthy diet and limiting screen time.
- Listen to your teacher or key worker. They have experience of getting thirty little people into school every day. Let them use their insider knowledge to get your child inside the building!
- Hold space for fears. Your child might be scared of being in a new place, being away from you, not knowing how they will be looked after, not knowing where things are. You want to show you are listening, and that you can reassuringly think of solutions to meet any issues that arise.
- Hold space for irregular behaviour. We all behave differently in the face of change. You may see a clingy, sad and exhausted little child or a moody, angry one, throwing things around – or even one who is withdrawn and silent. All are a sign of change and the impact on the body and brain. Remember, your child is not consciously choosing to behave like this!

Firework idea

In recent years, as an alternative to shouting at your child if they don't want to leave the park or play date, many parents will pretend to leave as a way to force their child to move. It seems harmless but it is inherently setting up the idea that the parent would leave their child in a public place if they were running late. That cannot make children feel safe. Try to think of other ways to move your child on to the next activity, like adding fun or connection by suggesting a race or a piggy back.

For Children Older Than Five

If your child develops separation anxiety at a later stage, consider:

- What has been going on in your family in the last six months? Illness, death, divorce, moving house, big changes? Has anything come up at school? Friendship issues, angry teachers, difficult work?
- What fears have come up because of it?
- If they were to stay with you instead of being at school, what would be different?
- If they were to stay with you instead of being at school, what would they find out?
- Which bit of safety or information do they think they would get from staying with you?

- How can you make them feel safe without you?
- Is there an adult they can connect with at school?
- Are they worried about you? Do they want to stay with you to check you are OK?

If you have worked out the answer from these questions, you are aiming to show your child:

- They are safe at home AND at school.
- You are in charge of them; they are not in charge of you.
- You are sensible and can find a plan to help them manage.
- They can say what they feel and you will address it.
- School can be a safe haven to digest what is going on at home if we allow school to support us and our child.
- If there is a school issue, you will put social or academic structures in place to handle the situation.

Firework idea

If you have more than one child, make a special time each week or two to spend with each child alone. It doesn't have to be an outing. Set up one breakfast table in the kitchen and one in the living room and eat the same cereal in two teams, one parent with one child and the other with their sibling(s). Find a different day to swap so each child gets a turn with each parent. If parenting alone, give one child a special, focused evening with you where they can have a later bedtime once a month.

When to reach out for additional support

Consider looking for therapeutic support when:

- The child's separation anxiety has lasted longer than two months.
- They talk about or begin to refuse to go to school.
- The child has regular panic attacks.
- The school seems to be (accidentally) making it worse.
- They begin to panic in other places whether you are there or not.

Books to help your child with separation anxiety		
Children	**Teens**	**Adults**
The Invisible String by Patrice Karst	The Anxiety Survival Guide for Teens by Jennifer Shannon	Separation Anxiety in Children and Adolescents: An Individualized Approach to Assessment and Treatment by Andrew R. Eisen
In My Heart by Mackenzie Porter	Outsmarting Worry: An Older Kid's Guide to Managing Anxiety by Dawn Huebner	Everyday Parenting with Security and Love by Kim S. Golding
The Kissing Hand by Audrey Penn		
No Matter What by Debi Gliori	Anxiety . . . I'm So Done with You: A Teen's Guide to Ditching Toxic Stress and Hardwiring Your Brain for Happiness by Jodi Aman	
I'll Always Come Back to You by Carmen Tafolla		
What to Do When You Don't Want to Be Apart: A Kid's Guide to Overcoming Separation Anxiety by Kristen Lavallee		

Six

Help! My Child's Bedtime Anxiety is Giving Me Anxiety!

What are the very real fears hiding behind this anxiety?

- The fear something bad will happen and no one will be there to help you.
- The fear unsafe things happen in the night.
- The fear darkness will make it harder to find what you need or escape.
- The fear that your parents will not come back in the morning.

From the moment I met Estelle, mum to eight-year-old Leyla, I could see how hard she was trying to be a perfect parent. Leyla was her only child and she had given up work in the city to care for her. Estelle got in contact with me when Leyla began having panic attacks at bedtime. She would wake frequently and was very scared of noises in the night. Estelle let me know all the thoughtful things she was doing for Leyla and told me how she was focused on helping her in any way she could. She almost seemed to be looking for my approval. She was so anxious about Leyla, it was as if she needed me to tell her she was doing her very best.

Leyla was enrolled in a large number of extracurricular activities. Estelle would say, 'Leyla has had the most amazing day. She won the school prize for her poem about Frida Kahlo, and she won the chess club prize. After school, she went to her Japanese lesson then we went to have our nails done while doing our gratitude journal, then she did her silent reading while I made dinner. She was all smiles but then as soon as we got into her bedroom after the bath, she began to freak out.'

Estelle would proudly talk about her special 'Chat des Copines' idea ('copines' is French for girlie friends) – a ten-minute chat she and Leyla had before bed. It always started off well, but then Leyla would start crying and struggle to breathe as she had a panic attack.

When Estelle brought Leyla for her session, I found that if I asked Leyla a question, Estelle always answered. If I asked Leyla about her school, Estelle would say, 'She loves her school, don't you, Leyla? Her teacher is great and she has so many friends.' Eventually, I asked Estelle if she wouldn't mind popping out once Leyla was busy making things in my therapy room. Once her mother left, it became apparent that Leyla was facing all sorts of tricky problems. She told me the work at school was tiring and then the day didn't seem to end. She said she was always rushing. She told me she knew it was really important for her mum that she be constantly achieving and trying hard at everything she did. She did love some of her clubs and lessons, but there were lots she really didn't enjoy. I asked if she had told her mum any of these worries and she said that every time it got to the Chat des Copines, which was the perfect time to talk about it, she was so tired and worried about upsetting her mum that she felt she couldn't tell the truth. Leyla was holding in all her feelings all day, trying to do everything her mum wanted. The strain of pretending to be happy when she wasn't caused panic attacks, bad dreams and an overactive mind at night-time, leading to bedtime anxiety.

The work with this family happened in stages. First, with Leyla's permission, I was a careful spokesperson for her. I was able to say the things to Estelle that she hadn't been able to say. I showed Estelle that the pressure of her packed schedule, though well-intentioned, was troubling Leyla and playing heavily on her mind.

Next, we helped Estelle slow down and make space for her relationship with her daughter and their life together. The big change for her happened when I asked, 'What do you want Leyla to remember about her childhood? Time rushing to activities she doesn't enjoy and almost no time at home with you, or time where you were able to relax and enjoy yourselves together?'

Estelle simplified Leyla's schedule. She allowed her more time at home to relax in the evenings. She also moved the Chat des Copines earlier so there was time for Leyla to express her feelings before she had to lie down in bed.

After Estelle had made space for connection and relaxation, this quite speedily made bedtime calm and happy for Leyla.

Why is bedtime so difficult for children?

Bedtime is the only time children are expected to be alone.

Children are generally checked on and looked after by someone from the moment they wake up in the morning right through till bedtime. All through the day, parents, teachers, teaching assistants, school nurses and lunchtime helpers supervise and communicate with them. We send children a very clear message that they are not capable of being in charge of themselves.

When evening comes, we want children to stay alone for a minimum of ten hours. Some don't seem to notice the adjustment and are perfectly happy to go to bed alone and stay there till morning. Some are deeply affected by suddenly being expected to be alone for many hours. Faced with what feels to them like abandonment, their most primitive survival instincts kick in.

The feeling of being alone can make these children feel they could be in danger and they will have to deal with whatever the threat to their survival is all alone. It's hardly surprising they feel profound bedtime anxiety.

Their instinct that they are alone, unprotected in the dark and something bad might happen leads to hypervigilance. Their bodies are pumping with cortisol and adrenaline. We would say they are 'too wired' to fall asleep. They are hyper-sensitive to any sound or noise.

Bedtime is the quietest and slowest time of the day. Rushing and being busy distracts children from difficult feelings or worries. Bedtime may be the first time they stop, the first time they spend with their parent all day, or their first chance to think deeply and be alone with their thoughts and fears.

Our job is to make space for relaxation, expression and connection throughout the day so there isn't this explosion of thoughts, fears, worries and anxiety at night.

How to manage bedtime anxiety

Here are my ten top tips to try if your child suffers from this.

1. Reconsider Your Family Schedule

We tend to assume our youngest children should go to bed earliest. I often see clients whose older child is developing bedtime anxiety from being expected to play or read alone while their parent puts their younger sibling to bed. Think about making a change. Is there another way you could organise bedtime so that your most anxious child is not left alone? Could your younger child accompany you while you gently and slowly help your older child to go to bed without worry? Could you occupy and distract your anxious child with something connective (that links them to you), like making something for you, listening to one of your favourite stories from childhood or waiting for you in your bedroom?

Could everyone be in the same place for stories, calm yoga or cuddles?

Is it necessary for your anxious child to be alone at night? Think about whether it would help for them to share a bedroom with a sibling. Consider a virtual friend like a children's smart speaker to play a limited playlist of favourite songs or stories to soothe them to sleep once you have left the room. Consider a night-light, if darkness is an issue. Leave the door ajar or leave the light on outside the bedroom. Leave curtains a little open. Develop a going-to-sleep ritual: a spray of a night-time scent on the pillow, a little foot massage with scented oil, a sweet prayer or poem you always say to each other last thing at night.

Imagine yourself anxious and nervous, trying to settle to sleep. It's very tough. So finding lots of little ways to help your child stay calm and happy and to soothe the anxiety coursing through their body is the key here.

Firework idea

On your most stressful, jam-packed night of the week, start a Make Your Own Sandwich night. There's no cooking, limited cleaning, and children as young as two and a half can begin to make their own dinner!

To do it, just put out the bread and some filling options you know your child likes to eat and let them make their own sandwich then wash up the plate and knife. For them it will feel like a special treat. Dinner is fast, bedtime is earlier, there are no food disputes. What's more, choosing what you want to eat and preparing it yourself – even if you do choose jam and tuna sandwiches stuffed with raisins – builds a pleasing sense of autonomy and independence. You are three and a half and you have chosen your own menu, made your own dinner and done your own washing-up. You are skilled, competent and rocking out your very best life.

2. Improve Their Sleep Environment

- Help children feel calm in their bedroom. You could limit the activities they can do in their room by ensuring they do their homework downstairs, for example, to maintain a feeling of ease in the bedroom.
- Make sure the room is dark and cool.
- Let the child have input in how their room and bed look and feel – the feeling of bed sheets could cause sensory aggravation for some children, leading to additional stress.
- For younger children, designate a toy to be the night-time look-out. Explain the bear's job is to manage the night and keep them safe. Set it up in a good position so your child can see it from their bed.

- Get your children out of bed quickly in the morning and open the curtains to expose them to natural light or take them outside for natural light as early as possible. This will set up their circadian rhythm early so they sleep more soundly at night.

3. Make Time to Talk Earlier in the Day

Many parents use bedtime to debrief about the day with their child. It's quiet and it might be the first time all day they have been alone together. If children have anxiety or are working hard to mask their feelings, letting their worries out in one go at bedtime can cause stress all over again – as if they are still doing the scary test or facing the bully in class. It may feel counter-intuitive, but bedtime is the wrong time for a heart to heart. You want your child to be calm before they fall asleep, not re-live all the issues troubling them.

Make time for a chat earlier in the day. Include talking and thinking about things you are grateful for as part of the conversation whenever you can. Even a short talk can address and smooth over some of your child's 'big feelings' earlier in the day, making night-time less stressed and more comfortable for everyone.

If you don't have time for a full-on conversation, you can ask your child to draw you a picture or write a letter or a diary earlier in the day instead. Ask older children to check in by text or even with emojis!

4. Add Proprioceptive Steps to Your Bedtime Routine

For more information about this and a full list of ideas, see pages 102–105.

5. Make Home a Place to Relax

We are always rushing to get to school, work, clubs, swimming. At home, consciously stop the motion and slow the pace from time to time. Stop acting like a human alarm clock, hurrying your children from room to room, bath to supper and off to bed.

Think about what would feel calm for you. Time where it is quiet? Time outside? Time doing yoga or meditation? Time to cook? Time to talk? Time to read?

Show your children how to find joy in calmness. You may be upcycling a stool. You are listening to your favourite playlist while you do it. You are engrossed and absorbed. Your calmness encourages your children to find something equally fulfilling to soothe their spirits and have time to reflect.

Firework idea

If you are looking for quiet time for everyone from about six years old up, teach your children to FART! This is an idea from Australian parenting expert Steven Biddulph – the funny/rude name is enough to get most kids interested! The letters stand for:

- **Family**
- **Alone**
- **Reading**
- **Time**

Essentially it just means that each family member reads their own book quietly at a designated time. If you FART together even for ten minutes every so often, you will increase your child's calmness, concentration and capacity to find peace and enjoyment in books, something so many adults struggle with.

6. Make Sure Your Children Know Your Home is Safe

I regularly see children who are scared of the night-time noises in their home. Their night-time anxiety mixed with hypervigilance makes them feel in danger while alone in the dark. They can't sleep because they are listening out intently for what they fear are threatening or predatory sounds.

Ask your child to note what sort of time the noises were so you can try to identify them. Then tell your child the safety facts:

- Where we live everyone has to live in safe homes. It's the law.
- Homes make noises. The heating comes on to warm the flat for the morning. As the water in the radiator heats up or moves through the pipes to heat up the house, it

makes a bubbling hot water sound. That is the noise you can hear. When you hear it, be glad the heating is working and we won't wake up cold but all toasty and warm.

- The whistling noise is the air rushing down the chimney and coming out again. It's great because it brings us clean fresh air. There is space for wind to flow in but nothing else. (Until Christmas Eve magic happens – of course!)

- We lock the house up safely at night so no one we don't know or even do know can come in. Come with me and watch me lock the doors and windows.

- Any other noises you might hear are rain or wind outside, Mummy going to get water at bedtime or walking to the bathroom in the night.

- If there are any other surprising noises, Daddy and I will wake up and sort it out. We are in charge of the home noises. We are the grown-ups and we know how to keep our house and family safe. You do not need to worry about any of this or even think about it. That is our job and that's what parents are for.

Be specific. Give your child factual details about your home. When you hear a noise, it is our rattling window, the beautiful tree outside, the birds waking up, our boiler firing up. When the noises happen in the night, your child will now know exactly what they are.

7. Act as if You Have All the Time in the World

By bedtime most parents and children are tired out. We often want it to be over as quickly as possible so our children get a good night's sleep and we can go to bed or watch telly or finish our work. However, a child with bedtime anxiety is often most worried about the moment they will be left all alone.

If you are sitting by the bed waiting for your child to go to sleep, remember:

- The calmer and more relaxed you appear to be once the lights are off, the sooner your child will be asleep.
- Give them a little squeeze. Hold their hand or foot so they know you are still there in the dark.
- Get yourself some headphones, listen to a podcast or turn your phone light down and do something you need or want to do while you wait.
- Move your hand away a few minutes before you plan to leave so the change in pressure doesn't wake them up.
- Tell them you are happy to stay as long as they need you to and if you have to pop out to check something, you can always come back. (The feeling of relaxation flowing through your child when they realise you are not rushing off anywhere should help to make it the fastest bedtime ever.)
- If these changes do not instantly make bedtime quicker, it's because your child doesn't have enough experience of you staying calm till they fall asleep or coming back to check on them to be able to relax at bedtime. Be present.

Take your time. Build on your child's relief after several consecutive nights of reassurance. Once you have banked a few good examples of you doing what your child hopes you will at bedtime, you should find they are finally able to snuggle down calmly, relax and go to sleep.

The ideas above are not intended to be done forever. They are a stepping stone to a calmer bedtime which then leads to the likelihood that they will be able to put themselves to bed at a later date.

Firework idea

Have you heard of sleep nudging? It is the idea that we work out what the smallest steps are between where we are now and where we want to be, and slowly move through them, giving our child time to relax into each stage. For example, imagine we have a child who sits on our lap on a rocking chair until they fall asleep, but our goal is that eventually our child will lie down in bed alone to sleep independently.

- **Start: Rock in chair, move to bed, stay till child is fully asleep.**
- **Nudge 1: Parent starts bedtime lying next to the child in their bed, stay till they are fully asleep (two weeks).**
- **Nudge 2: Parent lies in bed, sings a set number of songs or reads a book, parent to then move out of**

the bed and sit on a chair until child falls asleep (two weeks).

- Nudge 3: Child lies in bed, parent sits on chair nearby waiting until child is asleep.
- Nudge 4: Child lies in bed with torch, parent reads one book and then gives child book and torch. Parent says they will be back, then leaves for a minute while child is reading in the dark. Parent comes in and out to check on child (two weeks).
- Nudge 5: Parent sets up bedtime, child has torch and two books. Child reads and turns off torch, parent checks in later (three weeks).
- End goal: Child puts themselves to bed.

You may choose smaller or different steps, but it helps children make night-time changes without leaving space for anxiety. Praise your child every step of the way and reward them with something nice when they reach the end goal! Try to start the sleep nudging when your child is in a calmer phase.

8. Carefully Consider Screen Usage

Ask yourself the following questions:

- When and how often are your children using electronic devices?
- What are they viewing?

- Is it age-appropriate and low-jeopardy?
- How loud, flashing or bright is it?
- Is it firing up their emotions, putting them on edge or calming them down?
- Do you know what they are watching?
- If, for example, they are viewing YouTube, how are you vetting the videos they see and the accounts they interact with?

If your answer is you are not and you don't know, it's time to take advice about being tech-savvy.

If you think about it, you will realise it is important to supervise your child's viewing. Saying you don't understand that sort of thing exposes your child to all sorts of unsuitable stimulation, worrying content and anxiety. Check out the NSPCC free online safety virtual workshop or the UK Safer Internet Centre resources for parents and give yourself the skills to keep your children safe online.

All screens should be switched off *at least* an hour before bedtime. There is more and more data proving the blue light, particularly from tablets and phones, decreases melatonin production (the brain chemical we need to fall asleep) and children sleep less well if they are exposed to blue light close to bedtime.

Ask yourself how your children are using their tech. Are they watching on tablets very close to their face? Are they watching alone? Are they watching with a clear end point that makes sense, e.g. just until dinner or bath time? Limit arguments and stress by making absolutely sure viewing is finite. There should be no occasions when screen time stretches endlessly.

Here are my top three tips for sensible screen time:

- Aim to use screen time to increase closeness by watching together on one central TV. Cuddle or sit close together to watch it and talk about what you see.
- Be aware of what your children are watching to be sure they are not scared or overwhelmed before bedtime. Check the content they are looking at is age-appropriate and not overstimulating. Make sure it doesn't contain shouting, scary or confusing ideas.
- Separate screens and bedtime by at least an hour.

Firework idea

Sometimes children who have bedtime anxiety can end up being counted out of social situations like sleepovers as both the parent and child can imagine all the problems that could come up at bedtime in a strange place. Why not try a 'sleep-under'? A sleep-under is where children go over to a friend or family member's house with all that they would for a sleepover: pyjamas, sweets and activities. They play, eat together, do all the fun things that you might do at a sleepover . . . except sleep! The plan agreed by both parents is that at 9 p.m. or whenever the fun is over, your child will be

> **picked up in their pyjamas with their teeth all brushed ready to go home and get straight into their own bed. Just as fun . . . none of the fear!**

9. Use Sound or Light to Fill the Dark

Consider adding a sound machine, a smart speaker or a light projector to make the bedroom more inviting.

If your child is particularly worried about noises in the house, a sound machine fills the room with white noise which could mask creaks, whistles and noises in the walls.

If your child struggles with overthinking at bedtime, a smart speaker playing relaxing music or an audiobook could help. Choose a book you have already read to be sure there are no worrying surprises or purposely choose something gentle for younger children to manage overstimulation.

10. Don't Negotiate With Monsters

I believe deeply in helping children feel less scared about scary things . . . *but* I don't believe in MONSTERS.

It is really important that we separate the fear of real and irrational things for our children. When something is a real fear – i.e. there is a possibility it could happen – we should work to make it less scary but not minimise it. A child who is scared of being left out, spiders or break-ins can be told how rare they are or shown how to manage their worries better, but crucially all those things are real and they might encounter them.

When a child is scared of something that isn't real, we don't entertain the idea. We say, 'That's not a real thing. It is from a TV programme or book. It was made up by a person for fun. It's not real.'

There is no such thing as monsters. We do not give them the time of day. We do not make monster spray, write a ghost a letter or set a trap for an angry pixie – all those things make it seem as if we believe in them enough to require us to fight back. Instead we calmly and firmly state that they do not exist, so we don't have to worry about it.

> **Firework idea**
>
> If you want a really good argument to manage monster anxiety for clever kids, you can say, 'Technology is so advanced now, they have motion sensors, infrared cameras, night vision, drones and much more. If monsters existed, someone would have got a picture by now. There is no proof that these creatures exist now or that they ever have.'

Let's talk about who sleeps where and why it matters

Living in the Western world, we are brought up to believe the goal is to buy a big enough house for every family member to have their own room. But it doesn't have to be this way. There are numerous studies on co-sleeping, bed sharing, room sharing and sleeping alone and the conclusion boils down to personal and societal preference.

- Co-sleeping studies showed, on average, children who co-sleep get more broken sleep but have a higher sensation of calmness and can have a strengthened parent–child bond.
- Sleeping with siblings or sharing a bedroom can have a positive impact on anxiety as having someone with them overnight subdues most fears for many children.
- Sleeping alone can benefit children, particularly if they are supported to fall asleep calmly with an adult present or independently. Solo sleeping builds emotional regulation skills and improves sleep.

If an older child who has always slept alone suddenly wants to sleep with you or for you to sleep with them, consider whether calmly giving them a week in your bed or letting them bunk in with a sibling might calm them down faster and get them back to their usual routine. If so, say yes! It's so much more satisfactory than a stand-off that leads to overstimulation and higher anxiety at bedtime for all.

Remember you can always try something new and if it doesn't work out or it is clearly leading to less sleep for you, your child or everyone else, you can always make a new plan.

Firework idea

If your child is a night-time waker and you see them regularly after midnight, it could be a sign they are anxious and are producing too much cortisol. Our bodies are meant to produce this hormone as part of our sleep routine; the additional cortisol is what stops our melatonin production overnight and then tells the brain it is time to wake up somewhere between 6–9 a.m. If your child is already overproducing cortisol in the day because they have been anxious over an extended period of time, when their brain adds in more to start the wake-up process, the high level of cortisol starts the process of waking them up much earlier. They may also be easier to wake as their night-time hypervigilance means they have less restful sleep. Work on calming down their body and restoring safety to see if you can manually stop night waking.

Books to help your child with bedtime anxiety		
Children	**Teens**	**Adults**
The Worry Tiger by Alexandra Page *Franklin in the Dark* by Paulette Bourgeois *The Dark* by Lemony Snicket *Can't You Sleep, Little Bear?* by Martin Waddell *What to Do When You Dread Your Bed* by Dawn Huebner	*Good Night to Your Fantastic Elastic Brain* by JoAnn Deak and Terrence Deak *The Insomnia Workbook for Teens: Skills to Help You Stop Stressing and Start Sleeping Better* by Michael A. Tompkins and Monique A. Tompkins *The Awesome Power of Sleep: How Sleep Super-Charges Your Teenage Brain* by Nicola Morgan	*Generation Sleepless: Why Teenagers Aren't Sleeping Enough, and How We Can Help Them* by Heather Turgeon and Julie Wright

Seven

Help! My Child's School Anxiety is Giving Me Anxiety!

We are told our school days are the best days of our lives, but for many of us, school days were troubling and difficult. We might have floundered academically or socially, had trouble fitting in or been bullied.

Our own experience of school shapes the way we manage our children's academic lives. If we struggled socially, we might focus on making play dates for our child. If we struggled with maths, we will do our best to stop our child falling behind.

Our response to our child's school life becomes complicated when it turns out they find the things hard that we found easy. If, for example, we were academic high-fliers and our child struggles academically, it is more of a stretch for us to find a solution to their problems.

Some parents breathe a sigh of relief when their child starts school. They can be guilt-free about leaving their child for the first time since they were born. It is a huge relief. As children legally have to attend school, parents don't have to wrestle with the feeling that they ought to be with their children so they can finally relax. Other parents are filled with anxiety at the thought of it. They worry their child will be at the mercy of other children, strict teachers and the exacting curriculum without their help.

Whatever your perspective as a parent, your child must go to school, so we want them to enjoy it and thrive. All children will have days when they don't want to go to school or feel upset about something that has happened there. You will know if your child's school anxiety is more concerning than a fleeting feeling that they don't fancy going in on a particular day.

This chapter addresses the four most anxiety-based issues children face during their education. It covers academic pressure, exam stress, friendship dilemmas and school refusal.

HELP! My child's ACADEMIC ANXIETY is giving me anxiety!

What are the very real fears hiding behind this anxiety?

- The fear you are less able and different from other children in a negative way.
- The fear you could disappoint your parent.
- The fear the care you will receive is conditional on performing to a certain standard.
- The fear everything will always be too difficult.
- The fear you will need to attain certain marks or prizes to be rewarded at school and at home.

Belle was a naturally clever child who worked hard to get into the local grammar school. Having found everything in primary school easy, she was shocked to be put into the lowest groups for English and maths at her new school. Just over halfway through Year 7, she came to me highly anxious but also very depressed. She had lost her ability to see herself as clever and capable.

We started with a series of big boosts!

First of all, we boosted her academic levels by arranging for her to have tutoring in the subjects she was struggling with.

We also boosted her mood by adding moments in the week she could look forward to – like cooking dinner one night a week with her dad, new gymnastics lessons with her best friend and in-school mentoring with a child in the year above.

We boosted communication by letting the school know she was losing confidence and seeing what support they could give.

And finally we boosted her self-esteem by finding other things she could be proud of in addition to her obvious hard work.

Let's talk about depression in childhood

When we talk about depression, we mean a depression or a decrease in the positive chemicals our brains make, which affects the way we feel.

The main positive chemicals we need to make us feel happy, positive, capable and loved are:

- Oxytocin: the love chemical. We get it from being with people we love and like and who love and like us. We also get it from playing with animals or sharing smiles, even with strangers. It makes us feel loved.
- Dopamine: the success/reward chemical. We get dopamine when we meet a challenge, are excited to do something or feel productive. It makes us feel capable and like we are winners.
- Serotonin: the mood stabiliser. Serotonin brings us back to an even mood when we have been 'heightened' in some way, whether good or bad.
- Endorphins: the exercise chemical. We get this feel-good chemical as a reward for moving our bodies.

Often brought on by a sad incident, depression can also be triggered by any extended time in which we experience those chemicals less often. For example, social isolation leads to less oxytocin, low grades or constantly finding the work difficult leads to less dopamine, low mood can lead to lower serotonin and less desire to move leads to fewer endorphins.

If a child is unhappy at school, a place where they spend most of the week, this can have a negative effect on the production of the chemicals needed to feel happy. Just as we might begin to feel less like going to work when we get a new boss we don't like, children can get stuck in a low chemical cycle.

Unlike clinical depression, where the depressed adult gets stuck in what feels like a deep well of sadness, numbness and isolation, children with depression are able to snap back to normal quickly with the right support. Aim to boost the chemicals they have been lacking by supporting them with the following:

- Help them feel loved and liked.
- Help them feel connected to others of their own age at school or outside.
- Show them you are actively listening and making a plan to help them.
- Add physical activity to their regular routine – find them a weekly activity they can enjoy which involves them moving vigorously.
- Help them to feel and see the good moments and enjoyable aspects of life.
- Add more positive experiences and tell them you are doing it because you can see they are having a rough time.

If your child's depression has immobilised them and it looks more similar to the depression we see in adults, take them to see your GP as soon as possible.

I see children of all academic abilities experiencing academic anxiety. If they are noticeably high achievers, they fear letting people down. If they are middle ability in their class, they can feel they are progressing too slowly and they often notice they are not being given the hardest work. If they are low ability, going to school is exhausting and everything is hard.

How do we help children manage academic anxiety?

Try the following ideas to support your child.

Teach Growth Mindset and Life Skills

We can boost a child's self-esteem by showing them that no one can be perfect at what they do straight away. For more information on this, see pages 95–7.

Help Children Find Their Flow

A flow activity is something that is so absorbing that when you are doing it, you are not aware of time passing because you are calm, focused and happy. If you're not sure what your child's flow activity is, think of things they can do for a long period of time without getting bored. For example, they might like to dance, draw, kick a ball against a wall or listen to music happily for hours on end.

Having something they love to do can give escape and respite to children who struggle with the pressures of school.

Firework idea

Did you know that doing a flow activity actually counts as a meditative practice? For both adults and children, engaging in such an activity creates a special chemical in the body called telomerase. This keeps our cells strong, making us less likely to get cancer and thus live longer. Now's the time to go out and find your flow!

Add Appropriate Supports for Your Child

When we hear children are anxious about school, we often assume that they will need either therapy or tutoring, but there are so many other ways we can support children (and their parents!) who are overly anxious in this environment.

To calm anxious children, try:

- Spending time outdoors or doing outdoor activities.
- Joining a mindfulness group.
- Journalling.
- Proprioceptive activities – hanging, swinging, pulling, being squashed, heavy work (see pages 102–105).
- Children's yoga, art classes, martial arts.

To help children feel skilled, offer:

- A life skills group.
- Handwriting support.
- A social skills group.
- Occupational therapy.

For other therapeutic support, try:

- Art, music or play therapy.
- Animal-assisted therapy.
- EFT tapping (see pages 45–6).

To find support for parents, look into:

- Parenting support phone calls.
- Family therapy.
- Couples therapy.
- Parenting courses or groups.

Speak With Your School

Your child will not be the first to struggle with work or pressure in school. The most valuable relationship you can form to support your child in their school years is with the school itself. Use a combination of their experience, your understanding of your own child and your gut feeling to work together to make a plan that covers your child's academic needs and emotional requirements.

Show Your Child Unconditional Care

When your child comes to you or you notice they may be struggling academically, aim to show them you care more about their wellbeing than their academic accomplishments. Do that by listening and empathising with their feelings first and making plans for tutoring or handwriting support afterwards.

Talk to your child and explain:

- You are so sorry they have been worrying about this alone.
- You are so pleased that now you can help them through their worries.
- You empathise with their feelings of being left out, exposed or worried.
- You understand how hard it has been to keep up/feel inadequate/worry all the time – let them tell you how they feel.
- Give similar examples from your childhood when you were anxious at school.
- Let them know you only care about helping them feel better. If you are putting pressure on them, you will try to take some off. If they can't do the classwork easily, you will support them until they understand the hard things.
- Ask what help they want to make school better.

Remember Your Child is *Not You!*

Whatever your child is going through and whether or not you experienced something similar during your own school days, your child is not you!

The main difference is that THEY have YOU in their corner, on their team and in their life forever! You are there, thinking, organising and caring for them, and your kindness, planning and love are a protective force to make these events small blips rather than speed bumps or holes.

Separate your story from theirs. Listen to them and love them whatever comes along.

Books to help your child with academic anxiety		
Children	**Teens**	**Adults**
Wemberly Worried by Kevin Henkes	*The Whatifs* by Emily Kilgore	*Stressed Out in School?: Learning to Deal with Academic Pressure* (Issues in Focus Today) by Stephanie Sammartino McPherson
Jimmy the Jittery Jitterbug by Sonica Ellis	*Pippa Potter President's Daughter: Pippa Speaks Up!* by Elizabeth James	
William, the What-if Wonder on his First Day of School by Carol Wulff	*The Summer of June* by Jamie Sumner	
100th Day Worries by Margery Cuyler	*The Teen Girl's Anxiety Survival Guide: Ten Ways to Conquer Anxiety and Feel Your Best* by Lucie Hemmen	
The Magical Yet by Angela DiTerlizzi		
Hey Warrior by Karen Young		

The Cloud by Hannah Cumming *Very First Questions and Answers: Why Do I Have to Go to School?* by Katie Daynes *Just Ask!: Be Different, Be Brave, Be You* by Sonia Sotomayor		

HELP! My child is BEING BULLIED and it's giving me anxiety!

What are the very real fears hiding behind this anxiety?

- The fear you will die from being hurt.
- The fear you will be ostracised.
- The fear you will never be liked or included again.
- The fear you are unlikeable or unlovable.
- The fear there is something wrong with you.
- The fear you have ruined your life trajectory by moving school, missing school or focusing on this issue.

Eleanor was not a girly girl. She mostly spent break times on the climbing frame hanging upside down and having a laugh, but when a new child arrived in her class and decreed all the girls needed to play cheerleaders or they were *boys*, she was very quickly ostracised. The other pupils began ganging up against her, chasing her, touching her possessions, sitting in her seat, calling her nasty nicknames and ignoring her when she spoke to them. School was no longer a safe place.

I have worked with many different schools to support children who feel they are being bullied.

As a parent in this situation, you need to establish:

- Is this an extended campaign against your child?
- Has the school listened to your perspective and taken your child's pain seriously?
- Can your child be supported to improve this situation?
- Do you trust the school to help your child?

For Eleanor's parents, the answers were becoming clear.

When I spoke with her parents and her school, it was apparent the school could not understand how deeply ostracised Eleanor had felt in such a short time. I asked for their support and booked a meeting with the head of pastoral care. She gave me a long list of the measures they had taken to help, but in the same week the bullying had escalated. The bullies locked Eleanor in a shed in the playground and spilled her water into her lunch on purpose. I calmly explained to the school that the fact this upsetting treatment had occurred at the same time as they were implementing their interventions meant the changes were not working.

The school's response to my polite assessment was shouting and hostility. They responded to Eleanor's parents the same way.

If you feel your child is being bullied and the school is listening, understanding and making worthwhile changes, your child is at the right school and you should see an improvement over time.

If, like Eleanor's parents, you are sure your child is being bullied, there is consistent escalation and you can see the impact on your child, but the school does not seem willing or able to make the right changes to support them, it may be time to consider asking for more extreme intervention, allowing your child time out of school to regulate and then eventually the correct decision may be to change school.

When I met Eleanor in person, she was noticeably hypervigilant and jumpy. She had spent two months constantly looking over her shoulder. She was almost at breaking point. Talking to her showed she was seriously struggling to cope. I agreed with her mum that it was time for her to change school.

Earlier in this chapter, I talked about depression in childhood as a reduction of chemicals. This depression was clearly evident in Eleanor. Her body had been on red alert from the combined overstimulation of adrenaline and cortisol (caused by fear) and maybe even oxytocin due to being the centre of attention. Now she was simply at home waiting for a new school place. There was no dopamine from school. Her lack of interaction with other children left her depressed and low.

While her parents found her a new school, she came in to see me during the school day and we had fun together. We talked, laughed and Eleanor clearly had a great time. My hope was that my care and regard for her would help alleviate some of the unkindness she had experienced. I am glad to say the plan was successful. She began to blossom and, even more importantly, relax.

We worked on her anxiety about going to a new school. Her primary fear after being badly bullied in her last school was that she would never be popular and always be a target for bullies. We discussed whether she should change to match other children's expectations or continue to be her real authentic self. We developed a new exercise routine to calm her down. We gave her an active focus (she was allowed to repaint and design her room) and we worked with the borough to find Eleanor a place at a more nurturing school.

I am delighted to say Eleanor has settled very happily at her new school, made friends and is now thriving.

How do we support our bullied child?

Try the following ideas to help your child if they are having a hard time with other kids at school.

Try to Form a Clear Picture of What is Going on

First establish if your child is actually being bullied. All children behave badly sometimes. Is what your child is going through just a couple of children being nasty as a one-off or are they enduring consistent hostility? If they are being bullied, the aggressive actions will be consistent and continuous and are likely to be very upsetting and anxiety-inducing.

Try to make a timeline of events. What happened? Where did it happen? Who was responsible? What time of day was it? Do this after school every day for a week or two to establish a pattern. Try to ask your child about it casually. If nothing bad has happened, they shouldn't feel under pressure to come up with something so you can write it down. Note any deterioration in your child's mood.

Words matter. We need to be sure exactly what has been said. If there is name-calling, bad language, or derogatory or racist terms have been used, write down the exact phrases if you can.

What do you know about the child or children involved? Have you heard that they have problems at home? Does your child lead a noticeably happier life than those children? Take a deep breath and ask yourself what you want? Do you want the other children to be punished or do you simply want your child to feel safe and happy again?

Consider the result you want in the tone of your planned interaction with the school. Will the school be more responsive to a worried or angry parent? Could you start worried, see what their response is then progress towards angry if you need to?

Take Your Child's Feelings Seriously and Deal With Them Kindly

Your child may come home and say they are being bullied. It may be quite obvious to you this was a one-off occurrence, or that the 'bad' words the other child used are not all that terrible after all. Don't trivialise your child's concerns. To you, this was a non-event, something to brush off and forget about, but today it is looming large in your child's thoughts, stirring up their survival brain chemicals and worrying them. It is your delicate job to validate their distress no matter how small the incident, without blowing it out of proportion.

Take what they say seriously. Acknowledge how upsetting the experience must have been. Then reassure them that you don't think it will happen again. Explain that everyone, even children, can have a bad day and say or do something they don't mean and are sorry for afterwards. Tell them the 'bad' words are hurtful, but might not be as nasty as they imagined. Stress that if anything similar happens again, they must tell the teacher and tell you after school. If nothing is done at school to stop it, reassure them you will personally go into school and deal with the problem.

The conversation might go something like this:

> Child: I'm being bullied and someone in my class told me I am stupid.

Parent: Oh my gosh, that's so rude, I'm so sorry someone said that to you. How did you feel about that?

Child: I cried. I hate them. I'm being bullied.

Parent: That does sound really bad. Has that happened before?

Child: No, just today.

Parent: That must have been such a shock. What was happening when they said that to you?

Child: We were both waiting to get into the music room and I sat down on the chair at the front and they said it.

Parent: That's not fair at all. I'm so sorry. I'll mention it to your teacher tomorrow morning and we can track it in case it happens again so we can look after you. Bullying is a big word that usually means that person keeps coming back again and again and being unkind. We can look out for it and see if they do it again before we decide if it is bullying. We will all watch their behaviour carefully. You are quite right; you shouldn't be spoken to like that. Keep your distance. Don't sit with or play with that child for a few days.

You are aiming to show your child you know it wasn't their fault but not to embarrass them for using the word 'bullying'. And you are explaining that your child does not have to put up with it while others upset them.

Firework idea

Teaching your children when they are young that they do not have to be friends with those who are unkind to them can be life-changing. If we teach our young children to respect themselves and take themselves away from those who upset them, we set the standard for the rest of their lives. They are less likely to fall in with the wrong crowd or stay with a boyfriend or girlfriend that doesn't treat them appropriately.

Help Stop Catastrophic Thinking or Mind Reading

CBT therapy helps us understand the ways we can make situations WORSE all by ourselves.

Catastrophic thinking involves your brain going straight into fast-forward mode and immediately assuming the worst outcome. For example, your boss says they want to speak to you and you immediately assume they are going to fire you. Catastrophising puts your body through unnecessary additional stress. You do not know what is going to happen. If you could manage to calm yourself and see that nothing bad has happened yet, you would have better resources to address what is really going on.

Mind reading happens when we guess or assume other people are thinking negative things about us. For example, 'He didn't say anything but his face told me he hated me.'

Being bullied is distressing. Our children can make the negative feelings even worse by projecting an even more unpleasant outcome in the future. They might think, for example, that because they weren't invited to one child's party, they will never be invited to a party again. This is catastrophic thinking. On the other hand, they might feel as if they know how other children will respond to them or think about them. This is mind reading.

When you notice your child doing either of those things, kindly and calmly let them know. Help them see the situation for what it is and keep the problem the right size.

Speak to Your Child's Teacher

Whether your child is just being sensitive or there is a bullying campaign against them, your first line of defence is always the class teacher. They are in school and can see what is happening.

Be clear about how big a problem you think it is and explain how upset your child is. Ask for information and updates on the teacher's plan to tackle the issue.

Making sure your child's teacher is looking out for potential bullying can be the first essential step to stopping the hostile behaviour escalating.

Work on Your Child Forming Other Friendships

Being bullied can leave children feeling friendless and believing they are bad or unappealing. They think it is their fault they are in this situation.

Make opportunities for them to have positive social experiences with other children. Try setting up social situations with:

- Children from the other class
- Cousins
- Neighbours
- Family friends
- Friends from clubs

Look into whether they can join a Scouts or Brownies group, or a sociable after-school activity such as a martial arts class.

Find a way to show your child that not all children will reject them and it is the bully who has a problem, not them, by helping them engage with other kind children.

Ask for In-school Interventions

When parents contact schools, they often tell me they want to support their child but don't know what to ask the school to do. Here are a few options to mention in emails or ask class teachers in person. Ask for two or three interventions and hope that something sticks and is helpful.

Minor interventions

- Changing carpet spaces.
- Changing table seats.
- Changing reading groups.
- Instigating 'circle time' in which the teacher could discuss social skills, go over rules, or play games and increase the positive feeling in the class.
- Forming small 'social groups' of up to six children, in which adults model taking turns and discuss better ways to deal with social or behavioural issues (this can also be a way to help a left-out child make friends with a new group of children).
- Arranging extra art groups to take children out of class.
- Helping to create a quieter learning environment.
- Allowing them to sit with a friend.
- Choosing someone to be with them at lunchtime.
- Giving them a lunchtime job inside the school.
- Teaching the whole class mindfulness or social skills.
- Asking for an in-school adult mentor.
- Asking for a place your child can go that is inside during break time.
- Asking if your child can be moved closer to the teacher.
- Asking the teacher to talk to the class about appropriate language to use in school.
- Asking the teacher to discuss 'roasting', 'teasing' and 'joking about others' and to make clear this behaviour will not be tolerated and any child who continues will be given a specific punishment.

Firework idea

Have a social walk-through with your child on the way to school. Ask your child to think of what they would like to do at break time and who they would like to do it with. Remind them to chat to that child early in the school day to lock it in place, taking the fear of loneliness or exclusion out of break times.

Major interventions

These should be used when there are persistent issues that do not seem to get better:

- Moving class.
- Spending half the day in another class.
- Enforcing a zone of separation.
- Giving the other child something else to do at break times for a week.
- Getting a doctor's letter saying your child will take some time off to recover.
- Moving year group for either child.
- Moving schools.
- If the bullying is violent, you should expect the school to separate the perpetrator either in school or by keeping them at home.

> **Firework idea**
>
> **Aim to secure a school place at a new school before you inform the school you plan to leave. This will give less time for your child to worry about the move and less time out of their normal schedule.**

Hold Firm Boundaries and Protect Your Child

If your school is not responding and the situation is getting worse, make sure you stand your ground. This may be the first time your child needs you to protect them from danger. They need to believe and see you will do all you can to keep them safe. Knowing you will not give up on them will cement your relationship and relieve some of their anxiety in this difficult situation.

Listen to Your Gut About Moving Class/School

If at any point you think the school are making light of violence or consistent abuse, I would consider you justified in taking a vote of no confidence in the school and its practices. I would consider giving your school a short window for improvement – such as two weeks or until the end of term – and then make your decision to change schools and take action.

Books to help your child with bullying anxiety		
Children	**Teens**	**Adults**
Buster the Bully by Maisha Oso and Craig Shuttlewood	*The Gray* by Chris Baron	*The Teacher's Guide to Resolving School Bullying* by Elizabeth Nassem
Big Red and The Little Bitty Wolf: A Story About Bullying by Jeanie Franz Ransom	*How to Be More Hedgehog* by Anne-Marie Conway	*Bullying: A Parent's Guide* by Jennifer Thomson
Chrysanthemum by Kevin Henkes	*The Night Bus Hero* by Onjali Q. Rauf	*Teen Mental Health in an Online World: Supporting Young People Around Their Use of Social Media, Apps, Gaming, Texting and the Rest* by Victoria Betton and James Woollard
The Invisible Boy by Trudy Ludwig	*Emmy Levels Up* by Helen Harvey	
The Recess Queen by Alexis O'Neill	*Staying Safe Online* by Louie Stowell	
Stick and Stone by Beth Ferry	*The Survival Guide To Bullying: Written By A Teen* by Aija Mayrock	*How to Stop Homophobic and Biphobic Bullying: a Practical Whole-School Approach* by Jonathan Charlesworth
Giraffe Is Left Out: A Book About Feeling Bullied (Behaviour Matters) by Sue Graves and Trevor Dunton	*Confessions of a Former Bully* by Trudy Ludwig	*Bully-Proof Kids* by Stella O'Malley
The Not-So-Friendly Friend: How to Set Boundaries for Healthy Friendships by Christina Furnival	*If This Were a Story* by Beth Turley	
Strictly No Elephants by Lisa Mantchev		

HELP! My child's EXAM ANXIETY is giving me anxiety!

What are the very real fears hiding behind this anxiety?

- The fear you could ruin your future security
- The fear you will disappoint your caregivers
- The fear you will be left behind by your social group
- The fear the care you receive is dependent on the outcome of your exams
- The fear you will be outed negatively as stupid or lesser

Mendi came to see me as he was beginning to panic in the run-up to his AS Levels. He told me he had expected to do really badly in his GCSEs but, to his surprise, he had received the third-best results in his entire school year. From that moment school, which had mainly been a place to hang out with friends, became a place where he may actually be able to meet his parents' high expectations and a chance to change his own life.

To support him, we found him an in-school mentor who met with him bi-weekly to check he was on track. I was his spokesperson to his parents and helped them understand the nuance of his fears and support him with sensitivity. Our work focused on the notion of being the architect in your own life and how there was no wrong answer, only opportunities to have an interesting and varied life. We talked about what he thought would make exams less worrying and we tried to put as many of those elements in place as we could. He did his exams in a smaller group but in a public place, he was given breaks to use his calming techniques and his mentor was there to meet him on the mornings of most of his exams. And that was enough . . . He smashed it and sailed off happily to university a year later, feeling powerful and excited.

How do we help children manage exam anxiety?

Try the following ideas to support your child.

Help Your Child Start Early and Work Smarter

Showing interest and kindness feels very different from panic, criticism and disappointment.

- Talk to your children regularly and with interest about their schoolwork and exam preparation.
- Offer specific supports like helping them timetable effectively, reminding them to find time for all their subjects, showing them how to cut their work into chunks, etc.
- Give them space to work but remind them you are here to help.

There will be some subjects your child has to learn about that you are an expert on, others that you hated at school and others that you don't care about. Find a way to be on your child's team or bring in experts for the subjects you can't help with.

Track Your Child's Mood

If you know your child has a tendency to low mood, panic, perfectionism, overthinking or loneliness, find a way to track their mood regularly.

- Have a check-in chat every few days.
- Ask them to send you an emoji that explains their mood.
- Ask them to send you a selfie with their face showing their mood.
- Have them score each week out of ten on a Friday.

These quick snapshots can give us a picture over time and let us know easily when our child may need us to give them more attention, one-on-one time, support or care.

Teach Calming Techniques

The earlier on in the exam year you teach children to use regulation techniques, the more chance they will have to get over the awkward part of trying something new and embed it as a habit.

Lots of calming techniques involve deep breathing – this is to tell the body it has time to relax and reassures us we are not in danger. Deep, slow breathing sends the opposite of a panic signal to our brains and helps bring on a feeling of real calm. Here are some easy techniques I recommend:

Box breathing

Find somewhere quiet to sit. Aim to shut your eyes or look down to limit your vision. Picture the image of a box or square to help you stay focused. Use the diagram below as reference then hold that image in mind as you breathe. Aim to do this for at least two minutes:

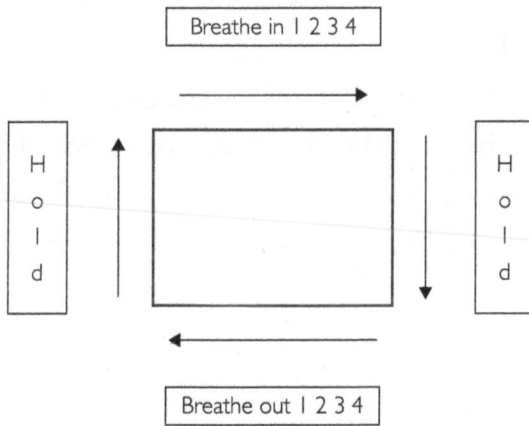

Bubble breathing

Sit somewhere quiet. Bring your hands together in a loose prayer position near your chest. As you breathe in, you can imagine that the air is blowing up a big bubble. Move your hands wider and smaller as you breathe in for five and out for six. You can also keep your hands still and imagine the bubble.

Body swinging

Other calming-down activities are centred around moving your body. This is regulating because we can remind ourselves to be in the moment and literally shake off the bad feelings. It also reminds our bodies to make more positive chemicals.

Try teaching your child how to do a full-body arm swing. This is a Kundalini yoga exercise where you start with your hands in the air with your arms straight above your head, then you breathe in and swing your arms down to the floor as you breathe out. You then fold at the waist, let your head hang towards the floor then swing back up. Do this ten times.

Arm swinging

A very easy and quick way to regulate your body is to perform arm swings. Stand up straight, relax your arms and then twist your body. Let your arms flail, keeping them loose. Let them hit your body. You can decide how much force to swing them with. Do this for about a minute.

Mindfulness practice or grounding

This is used to pull us back to the present rather than letting our fears take hold. If we focus on the here and now and see there is no immediate threat, our body will pump out fewer anxiety chemicals and let us do what we need to do without fear.

Try teaching your child this five senses check-in technique if they are feeling overwhelmed. Take deep breaths as you look around and find:

- Five things you can see – e.g. the floor tiles, your own hands, windows, desks
- Four things you can hear – e.g. children laughing, footsteps pounding on the floor in the corridor, birds outside the window
- Three things you can feel – e.g. the floor under your feet, the chair under your bum, the table under your hands
- Two things you can smell – e.g. shampoo from someone nearby, your own deodorant, flowers, cut grass
- One thing you can taste – e.g. toothpaste, breakfast, saliva

Body scan technique

Find a quiet place to sit or lie down. Take ten deep breaths into your stomach. Let your stomach inflate. It may help to put your hands on your ribs and belly as you do this.

As you keep your breath slow and steady, think about your toes. See how they feel in your shoes or socks. If you are sockless, are they cold? Can you feel the air? Do your feet feel tired, flexible or sore?

Move slowly up your body thinking about your ankles, calves, knees, thighs, pelvis, lower back, mid-back, shoulders, hands, wrists, elbows, neck, face and the crown of your head. Feel where you are tight or have tension and breathe deeply into those parts. Try imagining the worries hiding in those body parts, then imagine breathing them out in your out breaths until your body is empty of fear and full of light.

All these techniques can be used to add calm breaks for revision or before or even during an exam.

Speak to Your School

Schools may have a list of provisions or ideas for exam preparation and support for those with exam anxiety. They may have in-school therapy available or have a location outside the main exam room for children with anxiety.

Possible in-school options to ask for or suggest:

- Exam stress support group
- Exam skills reminder sessions
- A quiet location to sit the exam
- Stress management workshop
- Physical activities during exam period
- In-school mentoring
- Smaller groups for exams
- Being met by a friendly, known adult at school before exams

- Practising growth mindset as a school (see pages 95–6)
- Rearranging exam times if the schedule puts on too much pressure – you may need a doctor's note before asking for this

Show your child you take their fears seriously by helping them receive what they need to do their best.

Consider Using Affirmations With Your Child

Affirmations work on the principle that if we tell ourselves something often enough, we will grow to believe it. It takes on average sixty-six days to form a new habit or set up a new neuronal pathway in the brain. So, telling ourselves something that will make us feel more confident and safer could make a big difference in the run-up to an exam – but it has to be done regularly to make a difference.

Help your child to begin with these steps:

First, think of a time in your day where you could add a minute or two to say your affirmations. Then choose something to say to yourself. Pick something that is simple so you can easily remember it and repeat it each day. Think of between one and three statements that would make you feel empowered and safe. You can come up with your own or choose from the list below:

- I am safe.
- I am doing all I can.
- I can do anything I put my mind to.
- As I breathe, I breathe out stress.
- I have options for my life.
- My life will be an adventure.
- I will look back at my stress and smile.
- This too shall pass.
- I am in control of my thoughts and emotions.
- I am proud of myself.
- I am trying my best.
- I trust myself.

Once you have decided on your affirmations, find a quiet place and say them to yourself. Try to repeat each of your sentences at least ten times.

Best practice would be to do your affirmations in both the morning and evening. You can use them as part of a routine to stave off anxious feelings or even to find a sense of control in a more extreme anxiety attack.

Manage Anxious Feelings Using the Rain Strategy

RAIN stands for:

- R: Recognise
- A: Allow
- I: Investigate
- N: Nurture

This is a mindfulness practice that can help our children understand how they feel, give themselves compassion, meet their needs and move on. It can be done like this:

- **Recognise** the feeling you have; note the sensations in your body. If you feel anxious, is there a tightness to your chest, a buzzing in your stomach, do you feel hot? Note the feeling without judging whether or not what you feel is justified or fits to the situation. Just notice it.
- **Allow** yourself to feel that way; do not try to push it down, fix it quickly or ignore it. Allow the feeling to sit in your body for a few minutes before trying to stop it.
- **Investigate** gently with curiosity and kindness. Ask: what does this emotion want me to know about myself? What is making me feel this now? Begin making connections between feelings and thoughts. You might say, 'I know I am feeling so anxious about this exam because I feel it's an important part of my plan for the next few years. It's important to me and I don't want to hold myself back.'
- **Nurture** yourself by thinking about what you might need to manage this feeling and the emotions it creates. You may say, 'I think I should drink some water and also tell myself there are lots of routes to go where I want to go, the fastest may not be the best. I can only try my hardest and that's what I'm going to do.'

We may need to practise this method with our children the first few times, but once they get good at stopping, breathing and going through the steps, we will have helped them learn a very thoughtful and loving method to manage uncomfortable feelings that they can utilise for the rest of their lives.

Support Your Child in Their Fears and Feelings

Our children may just want to share how nervous they are without needing any other support. Our job is to hear them and believe how deeply they feel this. We can do that by listening as they speak and not interrupting. We should pretend we are at our child's feelings' press conference. Let them make their opening statement. Then ask questions that show you understand and care about their experience. Some of your questions should be to seek more detail; others can be supportive if needed.

Add Reality

It is true that exams are a big deal and can help your child decide on a path for the next few years, but there are other routes available to achieve your child's goals.

Remind your child:

- They will work hard and are likely to achieve the results they need.
- They can always retake any exams they are unhappy with.
- There's no one correct way to achieve anything in life.

- Whatever grade they achieve, you will help them get to their next step.
- If they are doing A-levels, explain that universities often take students with slightly lower grades anyway.
- Universities also offer clearing places for any courses that are not full. It's very easy to find a great place at an amazing university or college whatever your grades.

Learn the Best Exam Technique

Remind them of these skills:

- What is the question asking you to do?
- How many points is each question worth? Allocate your time accordingly.
- Practise past papers in exam conditions so you are not shocked by the time pressure.
- Practise in silence to make sure the quiet isn't a shock in the real thing.

Show Unconditional Love

Remind your children that whatever the result, you will love and support them. Explain the exam doesn't assess all the most special things about them – their kind heart, their amazing sense of humour, their quirky hobbies, their deep relationships. It tells us nothing about the person they are, only how well they do on tests.

Remind them you know they will try their best and that is all you can ask. You will like and love them no matter what.

> **Firework idea**
>
> **Add layers of confidence to your child's pre-exam routine. Help them do things to feel strong. Tell them to dress up in clothes that make them feel fantastic or help them boost their confidence by teaching them the dopamine-inducing, science-supported 'superhero stance' and reminding them to strike it. Remind them of a clever character from literature or film to focus on and embody.**

When and how to seek external support

Seek help if your child is constantly anxious and showing signs of:

- Panic attacks.
- Self-harm.
- Threatening or planning exam refusal.
- School refusal or sudden separation anxiety.
- Closing down and disengaging from school and/or other parts of life due to anxiety.

Consider how long it is until exams when choosing your intervention. If you've still got most of the year left before the exams, you can find an adolescent or young adult specialist therapist. Most will have had lots of experience supporting children through their final school years.

If there's only a few weeks until exams start, you can try the following for a short-term fix:

- Hypnotherapy.
- CBT (see page 41).
- EFT tapping (see pages 45–6).
- Guided meditation in person or online.
- A life coach.

Books to help your child with exam anxiety		
Children	**Teens**	**Adults**
Too Shy for Show and Tell by Beth Bracken *Jack's Worry* by Sam Zuppardi *The Big Test* by Julie Danneberg	*The Anti-Test Anxiety Society* by Julia Cook *The Perfectionism Workbook for Teens: Activities to Help You Reduce Anxiety and Get Things Done* by Ann Marie Dobosz *Say 'No' to Exam Stress: The Easy to Use Programme to Survive Exam Nerves* by Anthony James *The Teenage Guide to Stress* by Nicola Morgan	*Teenager Exam Stress: A Parents' Survival Guide: Stop Feeling Like a Failure and Learn How to Cope* by Linda Witchell
	Supporting Kids and Teens with Exam Stress in School: A Workbook by Joanne Steer	

HELP! My child is TOO ANXIOUS TO GO TO SCHOOL and it's giving me anxiety!

What is the fear hiding behind this anxiety?

- The fear school is a dangerous place.
- The fear that the school is not capable of looking after you.
- The fear you are different from other children.
- The fear you will never be able to attend school again.
- The fear you are disappointing your parents or caregiver.
- The fear everyone will give up on them.
- The fear you will not have a social life.

I met Luna (age ten) when I was called to her school to help support her. The first Covid-19 lockdown was over and most children had rushed back to school. Not Luna. Her dad told me she had seemed truly happy in lockdown. She had been frequently absent from school in 2019 and felt liberated when the pandemic allowed her to stay at home.

Luna was so distressed to be at school she could hardly enter the building. We even did two of our sessions in the school playground drawing on paper on the ground. Her dad would sit outside the school building for hours every day in his car waiting for the school to call and ask him to take her home. Sometimes, the call came at 9.20 a.m. after teachers had tried carrying her in, bribing her, using her best friend to walk her in or even letting her work in the school office all day.

Our sessions turned out to be the best way to get her into school. We laughed together, made messy crafts, wrote funny stories and designed our own games and, while she was busy, we talked. She talked about everything. She was very chatty and would bring things in from home to show me. Some weeks they were stickers or plastic animals. One week she brought in a photo of herself with her grandpa, who had died a few years earlier. She talked about him often.

In one of our sessions, she opened up about the last time she had seen him. She had gone to his house for a barbecue. He and her grandma were a great cooking team and they always invited Luna over at weekends.

On Sunday, the family had lunch together and then on Monday after school, they told her that her grandfather had sadly died.

To a six-and-a-half-year-old, it seemed that in the time it had taken her to go to school, her beloved grandfather had trans-formed from the smiling chef she was used to seeing to someone who had died and she would never see again. In just a few hours, he had gone from healthy and loving to dead. It was sudden and shocking and it had all happened in the short window while she was at school. I discovered that Luna's grief-stricken family had not thought to tell her when her grandfather was diagnosed with inoperable cancer and had been given just a few months to live. Her parents thought they were shielding her from the bad news. The barbecue was almost a year after that diagnosis and her grandpa had died in his own bed. Everyone in the family was expecting it, except Luna.

Luna now believed if she went into school, any of the people she loved could die suddenly. Once we worked this out, it was hardly surprising she couldn't bear to take the risk of going inside.

We invited her mum to come in to explain to Luna what had really happened in a clear but age-appropriate way. We worked on slowly extending Luna's school day by making quick check-in phone calls home. At first, calls home were made regularly. They tapered off as Luna began to trust that her presence at school had no bearing on her family's health. We made a big painting of her photograph of her grandpa and wrote letters and wishes to him. Her teacher chose a class topic that Luna really loved and knew a lot about and linked it to their literacy and maths so she felt like an expert in the room. We had therapy twice a week until she was calmer at school then we reduced it until she didn't need to attend.

Luna had a highly successful Year 6 and a smooth secondary school transition. I heard recently she is getting ready to choose her GCSEs and has been happily attending school ever since.

School refusal or Emotionally Based School Avoidance (EBSA) is one of the most difficult anxieties for a parent to face. This is because it stops your child from doing something they legally have to do and that all their peers are doing with ease. It makes you both stand out, and it stops you doing the things you need to do each day as you take your child back from school with you after drop-off.

Understanding the school avoidance cycle

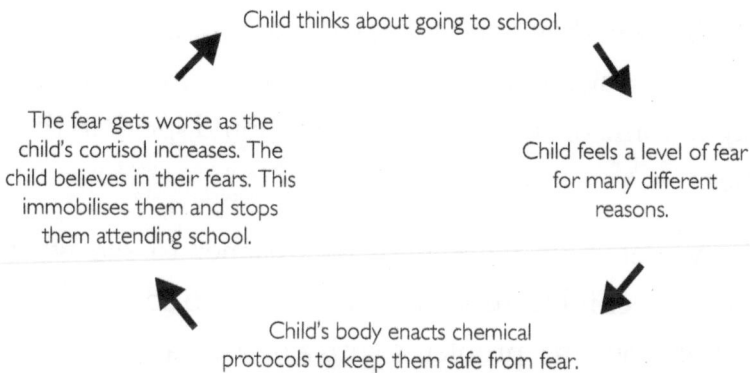

Child thinks about going to school.

The fear gets worse as the child's cortisol increases. The child believes in their fears. This immobilises them and stops them attending school.

Child feels a level of fear for many different reasons.

Child's body enacts chemical protocols to keep them safe from fear.

In the many cases of school avoidance I have worked with, both the parent and the child seem shocked by the scale of the negative reaction brought on by going to school. They have been caught off guard by how deeply they are gripped with fear, whether they know the cause or not.

The extreme nature of the fearful experience means the child doesn't have a chance to withstand the feeling of fear. They feel they cannot face it even for a short time. Then the continuation of the cycle means children embed their fears and believe them, which makes them even less likely to get back to school.

How can we combat school refusal?

Try the following ideas to help your child if they show signs of school refusal.

Speak to Your School as Soon as You See School Resistance

School resistance is very common. Every child will have days where they say they don't want to go to school. However, if it gets more consistent and they ask in a more impassioned way to stay at home or stay with you, you should speak to the class teacher.

Do some detective work with the teacher to see what has caused your child to resist school. Look into social problems, academic problems, problems with a particular adult working with your child. Did your child have an embarrassing moment at school? Are they bored, sad or lonely? Do they look or seem different from the other boys and girls in their class?

As a parent, you can also think about whether a problem at home is making your child want to stay away from school. Ask yourself the following questions:

- Have you or any close adults been unwell?
- Has anyone passed away?
- Have you had a new baby?
- Are you and your partner arguing more frequently?
- Are you moving house?

Consider the differences between school and home. Might the atmosphere be a problem? The work? How strict it is? Can you work out anything else that could be destabilising your child?

If you identify the issue, talk to your child's teacher and come up with a practical plan to make school more enjoyable and/or home more manageable.

If you cannot work out the reason your child is struggling, I would ask the school to:

- Greet them positively when they arrive.
- Have a chat with all staff working with your child, asking them to be extra supportive.
- Encourage your child socially.
- Give them any extra opportunities that crop up for a few weeks – sports fixtures, positions of responsibility, time out of class doing fun things – to make them feel special and included.

Try to Keep Your Child in the Same Schedule

I often speak to parents who suggest taking kids out of school as a response to bullying or other problems in school. What I see time and time again is that once children come out of the clear structure school creates, their symptoms and issues increase.

If we take anxious children out of school, we confirm their idea that school is not a safe place. It's a little like spraying 'monsters' with monster spray. It endorses and encourages their fears. Taking our children out of school shows them we agree they are not managed well at school, increasing their reluctance to attend.

Aim to keep your child in a regular school structure for as long as possible. Take them to school each day even if they only go in for one lesson and, if they're at home, make sure they work on similar things to their class at the same time so they don't fall behind.

Keep sending them to after-school clubs, particularly if they are also on the school site. You are trying to keep your child connected to the building and structures of school while you figure out and manage the causes of their refusal to attend. Send your child in to take part in their favourite lessons.

Try to show your child you support the school and think it is a safe place.

Firework idea

Aim to speak positively about your child's teacher, head teacher and school in front of them. The idea you think the school is incompetent or not listening will add to your child's anxiety about the school's ability to look after them. Vent to friends when your child is not in earshot.

Change Small Details

When your child begins to show increasing school anxiety, see if you can make small changes to keep them on track.

If you are usually late, arrive earlier to give your child time to warm up and get used to the environment. If you are always early, arrive later so drop-off is quicker and your child has less time to worry.

If you come into school through the playground, consider asking if your child can go in through the office or be met at the gate by a trusted member of staff instead.

If your school has a breakfast club or an after-school provision, extend or decrease your child's time in the building to see if starting or ending the day in a different way is enough to reassure them.

Other small changes to consider:

- Add a 'goodbye' ritual.
- Walk to school.
- Walk with friends.
- Drop siblings off in a different order.
- Let them walk in themselves from the gate.

We are aiming to take away chances for your child to be overwhelmed and, instead, to make them feel excited for the day. Shaking up the routine might be enough to re-establish a positive morning feeling.

Use Signposting to Boost Low Mood and Keep the Week Feeling Positive

When children are highly anxious about school, they cannot see all the good things going on. Make a timetable of the week and colour or highlight all their favourite bits.

Our brain has a section called the seeking circuit. It is in the middle part of the brain and it was evolutionarily designed to make sure we keep searching for better things. If the water dried up in the lake, the tribe would move on to find more water to drink rather than stay put. The same part of our brain lights up and gives us dopamine when we have something to look forward to. If we help our brains see the opportunities for positivity, it will boost our production of chemicals to decrease depressive symptoms. This can help to increase your child's positive feelings about the week and make it more manageable.

Firework idea

Ask if your teacher can find a special job for your child to do before school, like setting up the projector for assembly, delivering the registers or photocopying in the office. This sets up an opportunity to incentivise coming in early and producing dopamine earlier in the day.

Do Not Punish Setbacks

When our children are paralysed by a fear, particularly of doing something they have to do or did for years with no problem, like school refusal, parents can find this behaviour worrying, infuriating and embarrassing.

Suddenly we are faced with organising the logistics of working with a child at home, managing an overwhelmed and overly emotional child, working with a school and feeling frustrated or powerless. This can cause us to feel stress and anger.

However, it is important to remember the reason we are in this situation is because our child is struggling more than anyone can imagine. I have seen so many children cry and shout because what they want to do most is to go to school, be with their friends, feel normal and do what their parents want them to do – but they *can't*.

If you punish your child, you will only add to their feeling of being misunderstood. You are aiming to help them feel looked after, calm and well managed, and that you are on their team.

They cannot stop feeling this way without help. You are that help.

Work Out Misconceptions

In transactional analysis, the theory of 'eating a sandwich with the wrapper on' gives us a visual picture to understand how, when swallowing something with misconceptions or misunderstandings, it can get stuck in our body and it will not digest or pass through us.

With Luna in the story above, she had 'eaten the sandwich with the wrapper on' in her misunderstanding of her grandfather's passing.

With school refusers, we can often unearth a fundamental misunderstanding that is obstructing their experience of school. These are some common misunderstandings:

- If I leave the house, something bad will happen.
- If I go to school, something bad will happen.
- I made a mistake that no one will forgive me for.
- I have no friends and will not find any more.
- The adults at school do not like me and I won't be able to change their opinion.
- I have needs that this school cannot meet.
- There is something wrong with me that no one can fix.
- My parent has told me I go to a bad school, they will not be able to look after me.
- I am stupid and will never be able to do the things I need to do at this school.

Ask your child questions related to the most likely misconceptions:

- 'What is different about the way they look after you at school compared to here at home?'

- 'When children are badly behaved in your class, what do the adults do about it?'
- 'What happens when people make mistakes in your school?'
- 'What happens to people who fail exams?'
- 'What do you think you miss at home when you are at school?'
- 'Do you ever worry about me or anyone else in our family when you are at school?'
- 'Has anything changed in your friendship group recently that is worrying you about school?'
- 'Has the work or expectation of how much work gets done each day got harder or increased in this last school year? Is it all more difficult than before?'

If they respond to any of these questions with new information, you can match it to a misconception above and give facts and reassurance that the fear is not true. Then you can work with the school or work on what you are doing at home to alleviate them of the larger worry.

Take Your Child's Fears Seriously

I have worked with children whose school anxiety peaks at the front gate or as they enter the building. They feel as if a lion is waiting on the inside to eat them up for dinner. Telling them lions are in cages at the zoo and there are none here is not enough to persuade them to walk through the door.

If you understand your child feels this fear deeply, you can work together from a place of understanding and kindness to help them bypass and manage their feeling.

If you felt really scared of a spider, a person or a place, how would you want someone to help you? Would you want to hold hands as you entered? Be allowed to run away? Do the scary thing at a time or in a place where others cannot spectate?

The best way to try out the options will be on a day where you and your child have the biggest window of tolerance (see pages 63–4). Make sure you have both slept and eaten before you start the plan. Signpost your child to other good things coming that day.

When you think of a way to get your child through the scary gates, you can show them how proud of them you are for facing their fear.

Start counting positive outcomes. Telling your child how many times they successfully managed to face their fear, even for a few minutes, can inform their body that the thing they are scared of is not as scary as they thought. You will decrease your child's anxiety as you praise them and notice how well they have managed to do something they didn't think they'd be able to do.

Think About Your Child's Push and Pull Factors

In a school avoidance context, 'pull factors' are feelings, ideas, events and people that pull them towards school. 'Push factors' are the feelings, ideas, events and people that push them away from school.

You can look at the factors that are influencing your child to go to school or stay at home. Once you have a list of the problems and positives impacting them, you can aim to fight against the push factors and get them back into school.

Pull factors – towards school

- Being with friends.
- Enjoying learning.
- Enjoying sports.
- Having good relationships with teachers and staff.
- Feeling like you belong.
- Feeling well looked after and supported.
- Being able to let parents work and earn money.
- Being motivated to achieve and do well.
- Being 'normal' like the other children who go to school.
- Knowing you have skills to manage yourself even if you are having a tricky day.
- Enjoying the food at school and finding eating at school and breaks fun.
- Knowing if you find something difficult, upsetting or scary while at school, someone will help you.

Pull factors – towards home

- Being bullied or excluded.
- Finding work too difficult.
- Feeling academic pressure.
- Feeling stupid or incapable.
- Hating a certain lesson or member or staff.
- Feeling pressure to perform in competitive sport.
- Feeling that adults at school do not like you or think you are bad.
- Feeling ignored or unnoticed.
- Wishing you could stay at home to be with a parent.
- No motivation to learn.
- Low expectations for yourself or your life.
- Knowing your parent is unwell and needs help or could have an emergency while you are out of the house.
- Feeling embarrassed and awkward about missing school and not wanting to have to explain yourself.
- Feeling sad and depressed after a divorce, bereavement or life change and wanting to stay at home as you are lacking energy, confused and don't want to cry at school.
- Feeling fearful you will become overwhelmed by a sensory overload at school: too loud, too close to others, too much.
- Finding the food at school unappetising or scary.
- Feeling fearful you will let your parents down.
- Feeling scared you will be told off or punished for your behaviour.

- Feeling self-conscious, pressured or overwhelmed by eating in public.
- Feeling that school is not a safe place.
- Feeling that if you have a problem at school no one will help you.

Think about which factors sound like they apply to your child. Make a list of their pull and push factors.

Consider which factors are logistical and can be sorted with organisation, such as providing them with a packed lunch, social support or showing them you are well cared for while they are at school and letting them know who will pick them up if you are unavailable. Think about which factors the school can focus on combatting and which you need to talk through with your child at home.

Think about how you can change pushes to pulls or just add in more pulls, like having a special job to do at school, being brought into school community activities by adults, or adding something exciting into the routine like being able to walk to school with a friend.

Consider Adding Professional Help to Your Team

If you have tried your school's suggestions for a few weeks and are still experiencing problems getting your child into class, it could be time to speak to other professionals and see if you are missing something.

Having a therapist, psychologist, psychiatrist or occupational therapist on your team can add fresh eyes to a problem when you are exhausted. A new perspective can help you to make better plans and get your child back into school.

Let's talk about when you should consider changing your child's school

To decide if a school change could be useful, answer these questions:

- Is your child's anxiety clearly related to an in-school incident?
- Does the school want to handle this very differently to you?
- Have you lost trust in the school and their ability to manage your child?
- Can you be sure it is worth the upheaval at this point in your child's school career?
- Have you exhausted the most obvious options at this school?

If you think the school has contributed to the changes in your child's ability to go to school and has not supported your family in a safe or fair way to help them back, it might be time for a change.

Remember, changing school can often be a long process. There may not be an available place near your home.

Taking your child out of school to wait for a place at a new school is confusing. You have worked so hard to get them to go to school and now you seem to have changed your mind. So changing schools should really be a last resort after all other options have been exhausted, and you should aim to have a place in a new school lined up before you withdraw your child from their previous school.

What therapeutic options are available for school refusal and anxiety?

All talking therapies can be helpful in this situation, as well as:

- Hypnotherapy.
- EFT tapping.
- Mentoring.
- Life coaching.
- Eye movement desensitisation and reprocessing (EMDR). EMDR is a therapeutic technique in which you follow lights with your eyes and tap your body with your hands while you talk about scary or difficult things that have happened to you. The idea is it helps your brain change the memory from something that makes you feel scared, worried or upset to something that feels less powerful and impactful. It can be done as a short-term intervention or

as part of long-term therapy. It can be a faster way to move on from traumatic events.

- Online support, e.g. notfineinschool.co.uk, https://school-refusal.co.uk/

You could also consider speaking to your local authority to see what other support they have available for school refusers.

What can I do if I can't get my child to school?

If you've exhausted all your options and you really can't get your child back into school, speak to your school and your local authority. They will provide support.

In more complex cases, you may be able to agree what is called a 'parent contract' with the borough, which states that you are not condoning your child's school absence and you are working as hard as you can to get them back into school. It is not legally binding, but it can enable you to put a clear plan in place that is facilitated by school, home and other local provision.

When should I consider medication for my school refuser?

If your child is showing panic and extreme anxiety in attending school for over two months, I would consider speaking to your GP to see if they can make a referral to a psychiatrist.

The medications used for anxious children are safe and administered by trained professionals. If it is clear that your child's anxiety has stopped them from entering the school building and they are regularly absent because of it, medication could be an option.

Books to help your school refuser		
Children	**Teens**	**Adults**
The Sunday Blues by Neal Layton *The Colour Monster Goes to School* by Anna Llenas *Very First Questions and Answers Why Do I Have to Go to School?* by Katie Daynes and Marta Alvarez Miguens *Angel's Brave School Day: A Story of School Anxiety Management* by Mark Taylor	*Can't Not Won't* by Eliza Fricker	*Getting Your Child to Say 'Yes' to School: A Guide for Parents of Youth With School Refusal Behavior* by Christopher Kearney *Understanding School Refusal: A Handbook for Professionals in Education, Health and Social Care* by Karen J. Grandison, Louise De-Hayes and M. S. Thambirajah *A Different Way to Learn: Neurodiversity and Self-Directed Education* by Naomi Fisher *Emotionally Based School Avoidance: A Compassionate and Supportive Toolkit for You and Your Child* by Dr Claire Stubbs

Eight

Help! My Child's Social Anxiety is Giving Me Anxiety!

What are the very real fears hiding behind this anxiety?

- The fear you will be left alone.
- The fear you are different from other children in a negative way.
- The fear you will never be able to find a group of friends again.
- The fear you are missing out on what everyone else has.
- The fear no one will understand you.
- The fear you will not have a social life.

Socialising is imperative for survival. In evolutionary terms, human beings worked out it was safer to live in packs and that there were many benefits to mixing with other people. Living with others would protect humans against predators. We could warn one another, escape together or work to stop the predator together.

It also provided a variety of resources, which still holds true today. Just as having hunters and gatherers in your tribe meant you would get more of the things you would need, we now get a variety of experiences, skills, personalities and activities depending on whom we spend time with.

Being with others also provides the chance for chemical inter-actions. The connection between two people who like each other makes our brains pump the chemical oxytocin, making us feel wanted, happy and calm. Being with others exposes us to diverse experiences which encourage our brains to create even more chemicals that make us feel good: dopamine, endor-phins, serotonin, brain-derived neurotropic factor (BDNF) and gamma-aminobutyric acid (GABA). BDNF is seen as a 'brain fertiliser' as it helps us make the best environment in our brains for learning new things and maintaining a healthy brain, and GABA is a chemical that slows down the messages the brain is receiving, which makes us feel calm but happy. We make this chemical when we play games with rules, for example, as we are focusing on the game, we know what the people around us are doing and we can forget what else is going on.

We are biologically wired to know we need to make relationships – first our primary relationships with our par-ents and then further connections with family, friends and work colleagues. Even people who are naturally introverted, or those with a lower social tolerance, still need other people to be around them. We notice a change in our enjoyment of life and work if those social interactions decrease. If we liked our boss and she goes on maternity leave, work is less pleas-ant. If we have a close friend who lived with us and moves out, we will miss them, and the lack of positive chemicals we make in their company will cause a palpable difference in our mood.

Both children and adults feel the need for good relationships, which puts pressure on parents to help their children be social and on children to feel they are included and have access to the pleasure friendship brings to their lives.

Our ability to socialise is based on three main factors:

1. Social skills
2. Language skills
3. The people available to us in a social situation

Our children may have good reasons to find socialising difficult based on one or all of those areas.

We cannot choose who will be in our child's class and whether they are nice, friendly children who will like them, but we can support our children with age-appropriate social development and help them grow and develop the language needed to make connections.

What are age-appropriate expectations for socialising and how can we support them?

Age	Social expectation	Language goals	First steps of support
0–2	**Parallel play** Children will play in the same space but alone. They may be aware of the other child and find it hard when they cross paths.	Children will mostly communicate in single words like 'Mama', 'eat', 'ball'. Children will use around fifty words by the time they are two. Children will begin to put two words together like 'big car' at around two years old.	Spend time with other babies of a similar age. Read, sing and talk to your child regularly. As you go about your day, narrate what you are doing out loud, e.g. if you are cooking, talk through the steps so your child can hear you. Model language to your child. When they say something, add on an adjective, e.g. child says 'bear' and you would say, 'Yes, big bear!' Cuddle them and bring them close to you when they feel worried about something.
2–3	**Parallel play** continues Children will mostly play alone with similar items in a similar place.	Children will begin to make two-word sentences like 'eat biscuit'. Children will have a vocabulary of around 200–300 words.	Talk, read and sing to your child regularly. Find a nursery that prioritises children's emotional needs.

They now play with more awareness of others. They can be helped to do basic turn-taking but will struggle to share or play with others.	Children will begin to follow simple instructions like 'Stand up' or 'Give me the bear'. Children will start using question words like 'where?' and 'why?'	Give your nursery a glossary of sounds, noises or phrases your child makes and what they mean. Arrange play dates with children from and outside of nursery. If your child talks about a particular child, lean into the friendship and make contact with the parent. Practise turn-taking at home by playing games. Practise answering and asking questions – e.g. 'How was your day?' or 'What did you have for lunch?' – and then asking your child to ask you. Begin to teach certain independent skills if possible, like handwashing, safely walking up and down stairs. Notice if your child is nowhere near these goals and speak to your GP. Ask your nursery for a speech and language group or assessment if you are worried they are being hindered by low speech.

| 3–5 | **Associative play**
Children will still mostly play alone. They may begin to play in a similar way with those nearby, e.g. building blocks next to each other or digging in the same section of a sand pit.

Cooperative play
Children may begin to join in with one idea in play, like a role play, building something together or retelling a story. This will be much more likely with adult support. | Children will make three- or four-word sentences regularly.

They will use pronouns like 'me', 'you' and 'I'.

They will start to correctly use plurals like 'apples' or 'chairs'.

Family members or those who spend time regularly with the child will begin to understand most of what they say.

Children will recount events from the day with some accuracy. | If your child talks about a particular child, lean into the friendship and make contact with the parent.

Practise shared play at home, e.g. building together, doctors, simple games like 'I spy'.

Narrate how you play and explain your thinking in age-appropriate language, e.g. 'Next I'm going to check your temperature with the thermometer in your mouth, then I'm going to use the hammer to tap you on the knee and check your reflexes.'

Let children know they never have to be friends with anyone who isn't kind to them, hurts them or makes them feel uncomfortable.

Help them practise storytelling skills by talking about books you have read and the best and worst bits of the story. |

Age	Milestone	Goals	What you can do
			If your child wants to use their idea in play, support them and keep them on track.
			Begin to teach certain independent skills if possible, like getting dressed, cutting soft food with a children's knife, helping with laundry.
			Notice if your child is nowhere near these goals and speak to your GP.
			Ask your nursery for a speech and language group or assessment if need be.
5–7	**Cooperative play expands** Children can take on structured roles or play team games and will begin to be in charge of their own imaginative games.	Children will speak in full sentences. They will be understood by all who talk to them. They will use question words with ease.	Get children outside and moving as often as possible. Show children how to start a conversation by asking, 'What's your name? Do you want to play X with me?' Actively make play dates or social arrangements with families in your child's class.

Complex social interactions		
Children will begin to have more complex friendships.	They will understand and use the concept of a beginning, middle and end when they tell a story.	Lean into positive interactions your child talks about and invite that child over.
They will begin to care deeply for their friends and think about them when they are apart.	Vocabulary begins to grow and children will use more complex words often.	Let your child know they never have to be friends with anyone who isn't kind to them, hurts them or makes them feel uncomfortable.
They will begin to navigate minor conflict resolution alone.	They can follow directions with a few steps.	Tell age-appropriate jokes and show your child the funny games and school tricks you knew as a child.
	They will mostly speak in a grammatically correct way.	Talk to your child regularly.
	They will begin to understand jokes.	Eat meals at a table as a family as often as possible.
	They will be able to maintain a conversation with two or three back-and-forth responses.	When correcting children's speech mistakes, do it indirectly by repeating it correctly without pressure or shame, e.g. Child: 'Did I went to Grandma's house?' Parent: 'Yes, you did go to Grandma's house.'
		If your child is still hard to understand, consider speech therapy through your GP or privately.

7–10	**Team play**	Children will have an increased vocabulary, including more descriptive language.	Help your child find activities that they love.
	Children will enjoy organised sports and games.		Aim to find a mix of sporty and creative clubs.
	They will begin to understand the concept of teamwork.	They will be able to explain abstract concepts or ideas that are not literal or happening now to others.	Let your child know they never have to be friends with anyone who isn't kind to them, hurts them or makes them feel uncomfortable.
	Friendships become more significant.	They will be able to join in a more complex discussion.	
	Friend groups rather than best friends become more important.	They will be able to summarise something seen, heard or read.	Be aware of the social dynamics in your child's class and speak to the teacher if it doesn't seem right.
	Competitive play	They will begin to use persuasive language.	Help foster relationships with the whole group, not just one child.
	Children will begin to understand competition and its inner workings.		Involve your child in interesting and age-appropriate news stories or goings-on.
	They begin to get better at losing.		Consider some children will thrive when not loaded up with after-school activities. They may need time at home to relax.
	They are able to manage sportsmanship.		Help children find self-worth with roles and responsibility at home.

			Eat meals at a table as a family as often as possible. Aim to make time to spend with your child alone at least once a month. Stay interested: what are they watching, playing and reading? What do they like?
10–12	**Interest-based play** Children begin making friends primarily around shared interests. Peer interactions become more emotionally complicated. **Group activities** Children begin to find their strengths and talents in hobbies, clubs and sports. This leads to closer social relationships.	Children are able to report on what they have seen, done, heard or read with depth and accuracy. Children will begin to show a mastery in written communication. Children will use more complex speech structures regularly and with fluency.	Continue to help your child try out and find their interests. Find things they can achieve in but also enjoy. Be an available support for your child. Involve and engage them in age-appropriate stories and ideas. Talk to them and spend time with them doing things they love. Are there ways to help your child take on a more prominent social role if they wanted to, like letting them host a regular event at your house? Stay interested: what are they watching, playing and reading? What do they like?

12+		
Social play Friendships begin to take precedence over other activities. Play now changes to social gatherings and parties. Teens will bond over places where they have been together. **Exploration** Socialisation is used as a means to explore identity. They will try new things such as style, music and relationships to work out their identity. Children's new interests will regularly be introduced by peers, rather than school or home.	Children will begin to express and justify their own opinions. They will begin to understand when it's appropriate to use more formal language in person and in written work. Children will be able to display critical thinking skills and problem-solve independently.	Eat meals at a table as a family as often as possible. Be open with them about the changes in your relationship and what teenagers can be like. Take your children's social life seriously and help facilitate friendships that you can see are positive. Are there ways to help your child take on a more prominent social role if they want one, like hosting a regular event at your house? Be supportive of children exploring their identity; consider that your support will make each step an easier transition and make any change less of an act of rebellion. Speak openly about dating and how to be safe and value yourself. Stay interested: what are they watching, playing and reading? What do they like? Eat meals at a table as a family as often as possible.

Additional support for your children socially at any age

Age 0–5

Follow your child's lead

I have always said that shyer children are simply showing how intelligent they are! There are so many surprising and confusing things about the world that it makes sense that if you are clever, you realise it could be wise to hang back in a new setting and wait to see what unfolds before diving in.

Children (and adults) are allowed to be nervous. It's perfectly acceptable to take a little time to warm up and they are allowed to seem very fearful and then suddenly change their minds.

Our job is to calmly support them. There are no prizes for being the child holding the entertainer's hand at the front of the party one second after arrival. Parents must not think it gives a poor impression of them or their child if they want to stay at the back and observe.

The more we show our child we understand their hesitation and will be there to help them, the less there is for them to fear. It takes time and practice but that way we can support our children while they work out the rules and any surprises that are in store for them.

Do a situational walk-through

On your way to the party or play date, tell your child where you are going, what you know about it.

Tell them:

- Who will be there.
- How long you will be staying.
- What might happen there.
- If your child has had problems before with things like noise, a fear of joining a big group or being left somewhere, let them know what you are planning to do to improve that situation this time. For example, you might say, 'Last time we didn't love the noise at the party, so this time I think we could stand at the back until we are used to it.'
- If they don't like it, remember you can just go home!.

Give options on arrival

When you arrive at a party or play date, ask your child:

- 'Do you want to join the group or stay with me?'
- 'Would you like to go upstairs or play down here?'
- 'Do you want to eat something now or later?'

Offering children options gives them a sense of control and power even in moments in which they feel overwhelmed.

Use positive language to describe your child

If someone asks you why your child isn't joining in, try phrases like:

- 'He's just taking it all in first.'
- 'She just likes a minute to suss out the situation.'
- 'We always stay together at the beginning until we work out what's going on.'
- 'He's an observer first!'
- 'She's such a sensible girl, she's just waiting see what the rules of this place are.'

When we describe children as shy, this can become a label they have to work against, despite the fact that their behaviour is just a sensible method of working out a new place or situation. It can make them feel shame or embarrassment when arriving at a new place is already difficult.

Do not force children to share

One area children genuinely struggle with during play dates, even at their own home, is sharing. The reason why is that under-fives have very little understanding of object permanence.

Object permanence is the understanding that if you hide or can't see something, it will still exist. In children's developing brains, their inability to grasp this yet means that they will logically conclude that if you give something to someone, you have no idea if you will get it back.

If you are at your house, ask your child: 'Which toys would you like to put away and keep just for you and which do you not mind sharing?'

Then be respectful of what they have said and protect that boundary for your child. You can say things like: 'I'm so sorry, but Lucy just got that art set for her birthday and she isn't ready to share it. Maybe next time you come? But you can play with the ice-cream shop, the colours and the bears. Which would you like?'

This helps your child feel they have power in their own home and control of their own possessions.

You can also remind your child that their friends will not take home anything they play with. They will only use them at your house.

Teach language to help play

We can model social skills for our children when they are very young. We can show them how to ask someone their name and if they want to play, and how to explain our ideas clearly so others can join in.

Teach phrases like:

- 'What's your name?'
- 'Do you want to play with me?'
- 'Can I play with you?'

- 'My idea is . . .'
- 'If we play my game first, we can play your game next.'
- 'If we go on the swings now like you wanted, can we play in the sand next?'
- 'I want to play . . .'

Help your children practise saying these things at the park or during play dates.

Let them leave if they want to

If your child is distressed at a play date or party – remember you DO NOT have to be there. You can always leave. If your child is neurodivergent, particularly sensitive or just not enjoying it, consider the idea that taking them home because you saw they were unhappy or overwhelmed shows your child you care about how they feel more than the expectation that you stay at something until the end.

If you have to make an excuse, you can say something like your partner is locked out or you have to get back for a delivery you didn't know was coming. That way, you have respected your child's needs and met social expectations.

Your child may be in a phase where birthday parties are just too difficult to cope with. Stop going for a while and focus your energy and patience on the things they have no option but to attend, e.g. school, the doctor and the dentist.

Teach consent

From very early on, we can teach children consent in social situations. This means no one has to play a game they don't like and no one has to do something a friend suggests if it makes them feel uncomfortable.

Teaching children to say 'no' politely and helping them enforce their wishes will help them find more suitable friends and partners for life as they will learn to spend time with those who respect their needs.

This can also be taught through your actions. If your child says they don't want to be picked up and it is safe to keep them on the ground, put them down. If they don't enjoy a film, game, joke or song, don't make them participate. We empower our children to listen to their own feelings if we respond with kindness to their requests, so they will learn to respect their own wishes and the wishes of others as they grow.

Age 5–12

Use your social skills to support your child

When your child has a play date, imagine that the child is coming over to hang out with *you*! Help your child host them, set up activities and help them talk to each other. Model social skills and conversation by being part of the beginning of some of the activities. When they have a snack, sit at the table with them and engage them in conversation.

Saskia Joss

Show them how to say 'And you?' and how that continues the conversation.

Use role play to practise

Find opportunities to play role-playing games where one doll, figurine or character needs to find people to play with or needs to tell a friend they don't like what they do. You can practise asking clearly and asserting needs or ideas.

You can even say, 'I'll be Claire and you be you and you tell me you don't want to play on the swings!' and then swap roles to get it all bedded in.

Set fair social rules at home

Often, as parents, we choose rules that *our* parents insisted on when we were kids – or alternatively we might purposely set up the opposite structures to our childhood. Instead of copying your parents or deliberately doing something different as a reaction against them, personalise your rules to fit your family.

Start with rules about safety and build up rules that make everyone feel comfortable. Consider too how many of your family rules are just 'because I said so!' and not because they make sense.

Finally, keep in mind that many families will always fall on the side of their youngest child or their male or female child

223

if there is a sibling dispute. Try to strike a balance. Think about what you are telling your not-chosen child about their importance in your family and in the world. Should they expect that everyone will assume they are always right or always wrong? If you always champion your youngest child, try to see things from your older child's perspective. If you defend your daughter and never your son, try to break the cycle. Just because you are used to behaving that way doesn't mean you can't change.

Be a fair judge

When children argue or there is a problem, ask, 'What happened?' It allows a child the space to explain their reasoning behind their choices. Considering our child's reasoning even when we don't agree with it is empowering and helps children feel like they should be listened to and respected.

When we find our child doing something we do not like or do not expect, instead of asking 'Why?' we can try asking 'How come?' 'Why?' immediately implies we think what they are doing is wrong. 'Why are you in the kitchen?' makes it clear you don't want your child to be in the kitchen. 'How come you are in the kitchen?' gives the opportunity for their own ideas or reasons to come out. You can then move them or change the plan once you understand their thinking.

Help maintain social momentum

When your child comes home from school talking about fun they had with a new child, lean in and ask their parent for a play date or a meet-up at the local park after school. Help your child foster relationships with children they seem to get on with – it might become a pivotal friendship in the next few weeks, months or years.

> **Firework idea**
>
> **Some children struggle to play with others if their parents take charge of the play, so that the child is effectively a spectator. Try to hang back in the play and remember there is no right way to be a fairy, build Lego or paint a house unless it's unsafe. Empower your child to feel confident in their ideas socially by giving them some space to have them and then joining in yourself rather than being in charge.**

Speak kindly about your child's friends and their families

When your child has a friend over or you go with them to a friend's house, aim to keep criticisms of their home, the food they eat, the way they look or how they live out of your child's earshot.

Your opinion could stop your child making a connection or make them feel embarrassed to be their friend, making socialising even more difficult.

Age 12–18

Invest in your child's friendships

If we know who our child's friends are and are invested in their world, our children will be more likely to come to us if there are problems. Knowing the key players makes it easy for our kids to have a shorthand with us that translates easily into a comfortable relationship with us as they get older.

Help them work out if they are an introvert or an extrovert

We are all different and so are our children. Some people love socialising and being in big crowds and others do not. One way of thinking about it is to imagine that extroverts' emotional batteries get filled up by being with others and introverts are depleted from too much social contact.

We can help our children find friends and activities that help them feel happy, calm and fulfilled by noticing what happens to their bodies when they have been in a big group or with one friend, or what happens when they go to a quiet after-school activity compared to a loud one.

We need to help our children listen to the signs their body gives them about being with others and help them make a schedule that allows them to have friends and contact with others but not in a way that leaves them empty. If they are extrovert, we might need to give them more opportunities to socialise to prevent them from being lonely or in low mood without others.

Find things they love to do with an added social element

If your child is introverted or has become low or socially avoidant, work to find things they can do that they will enjoy where they will naturally be with others. If they love swimming, could they join a gym or a team? If they love art, could they join a local class, or if they are older could they get a job at a pottery café? If they like to watch sports or films, see if their school can set up a lunchtime film club. We know that even introverts can become depressed with too little human interaction and structure.

Have a family codeword

We know that peer pressure and doing things you may not feel comfortable with or are unsafe are issues that most teens will face. One way that we can counteract this possibility for our kids is to give them a codeword. This is a word to slip into a conversation with us that doesn't stand out but triggers them being picked up from anywhere they don't feel comfortable with, without showing themselves up in front of others. Set the rules around not using it for manageable problems, but if your child calls from a sleepover and slips in the word 'bananas' or 'quibble', then we will know they want to come home and we can show them we respect it by coming to pick them up, no questions asked. We will think of an excuse for them and get someone there ASAP! It takes the pressure off children to stick it out and see what happens when they have already worked out something seems off where they are. Get them out first then think of plans for next time later.

Think about your tone

There are lots of studies that suggest that children and teens are less able to listen when they hear a judgemental or lecturing tone. Children are less likely to take in information and more likely to be defensive when they think you are only talking to them to tell them what to do. If we want to help our children feel better in their friendship groups, get outside to boost their mood or help around the house, we will get much better results if we check our tone first and aim to be collaborative and empathetic.

Talk through safe and unsafe scenarios

As your child spends more time out of the house, explain to them what safe and unsafe socialising looks like. Set fair boundaries on drinking, sleeping out of the house and dating by being honest and realistic. Tell your child they can always blame things on you that they don't want to do. 'My parents would kill me if I came home drunk,' for example. Let them know that if they talk things through with you, you would always rather make it safer first than find out something dangerous or awful later on.

Listen without advice . . . until the very end

I have noticed the difference with younger children and teens is that when they want to tell you about something that has happened with friends, younger children are happy to hear what you think about their choices and answer questions as they go. Teens like to get it all out first!

Let your teen explain their side of the drama, sit back and listen positively as the soap opera unfolds and note your responses without sharing them. When they are finished, you can kindly let them know that calling their friend the B word or pretending they aren't having a party isn't the best idea. They know you are going to offer advice, that's why they are talking to you. Just give them a chance to express themselves properly before the problem-solving process starts.

How do you get through it as a parent?

Know Your Child is Not You

One thing parents really struggle with is when they are triggered to remember a feeling from their own past. The feelings of social pressure or isolation, not being invited to a party or being cheated on by a partner are strong ones – and the thought of these things happening to our children can make us panic. We know how bad it felt for us and naturally we want to protect them.

The thing is, they are protected because YOU are there for them.

Our children are not us. They are living in a different world and the care we have shown them and the resilience we have taught them will be the protective factors for their mental health over the rest of their life.

Understand Their Social Needs

The better we know our children and the more we talk to them and spend time with them, the more we can work out what support they will need to manage socially. This will help us help them whether they are sensitive, neurodivergent or confident. We can then add in structures at school and in other places to make sure they don't have to worry about the things we know they struggle with.

You Are the Coach Not the Player

The hardest thing about being a parent is not being able to step in for your child in difficult times. Think about the role of a coach, where they can help in training, share the experience and set up structures but can never step on the pitch. They have to let their players put what they have learned into practice themselves.

How can you make sure your child has been trained up for what the game of life will throw at them?

Firework idea

A study in 2009 found a clear correlation between young adults with social anxiety and those who had overprotective parents. To help empower your children and fight against this, show them how capable they are, boost them up – then give them space to show all they can do.

Breathe and Be There

Helping children manage socially is difficult for them and for us. It is important for them to know you will always be there no matter what, able to talk it through, reschedule, pick them up, find them the cool trainers or cuddle them and get out the house together after a break-up. We can be the safe house they come back to. Now all we need to do is breathe deeply and be pleased we have done enough to make it safe enough for them to come home to us.

What support is available for children struggling with severe social anxiety?

If you feel you need to take additional steps to support your child socially, speak to your GP, your child's school or search online for specialists in your area.

- Cognitive behavioural therapy (CBT) is a highly practical short-term therapy that helps children think through their coping strategies and then sets practical tips for getting past problem areas in their lives.
- Exposure therapy finds ways to gradually expose people to their fears and help them get used to the discomfort and difficult feelings that come up.
- Art and play therapy is the most popular kind of therapy for children. It allows children to use art or imaginative play to help them express their anxieties.
- Family therapy helps families function better and supports children through difficulties.
- Psychiatry is available for children who are too fearful to function in their normal structure. Usually a child will visit a psychiatrist to get medication for anxiety or depression when nothing else is working. It will normally only be prescribed in addition to therapy or counselling.
- Hypnotherapy can help children manage anxiety in a different way and help them regain control and calm.

Books to help your child with social anxiety		
Children	Teens	Adults
Too Shy for Show and Tell by Beth Bracken	*Ella on the Outside* by Cath Howe	*Why Will No One Play With Me?: The Play Better Plan to Help Kids Make Friends and Thrive* by Caroline Maguire
Brave Every Day by Trudy Ludwig	*Hey Warrior* by Karen Young	
Invisible Isabel by Sally J. Pla		

Shy and Mighty: Your Shyness is a Superpower by Nadia Finer *Behaviour Matters: Turtle Comes Out of Her Shell: A Book About Feeling Shy* by Sue Graves *Meesha Makes Friends* by Tom Percival *The New Social Story Book: Over 150 Social Stories That Teach Everyday Social Skills to Children and Adults with Autism and Their Peers* by Carol Gray	*The Shyness and Social Anxiety Workbook for Teens: How to Be Yourself: Quiet Your Inner Critic and Rise Above Social Anxiety* by Ellen Hendrikson *CBT and ACT Skills to Help You Build Social Confidence* by Jennifer Shannon *Rewire Your Anxious Brain for Teens: Using CBT, Neuroscience, and Mindfulness to Help You End Anxiety, Panic, and Worry* by Debra Kissen, Ashley D. Kendall, Michelle Lozano and Micah Ioffe	*Raising the Shy Child: A Parent's Guide to Social Anxiety: Advice for Helping Kids Make Friends, Speak Up, and Stop Worrying* by Christine Fonseca

Nine

Help! My Child's Anxiety About Death is Giving Me Anxiety!

What are the very real fears hiding behind this anxiety?

- The fear you could die.
- The fear you could be left alone.
- The fear you will not be looked after.
- The fear no one will fully understand you again.
- The fear you could also be unwell.
- The fear the world is not safe.

Jeremy (8) and Salah (8), best friends for years, had been completely carefree, gone on adventures together and were growing into delightful young men when an awful and unexpected event happened: Jeremy's father died after a short battle with cancer. His death was sudden and shocking. A few months later, I heard from Salah's mum. Her once cheerful, adventurous boy had become completely focused on death. He wouldn't sleep unless he could lie in his parents' bed touching them. He could rarely leave the house even to go to school. He had lost weight and had no energy. He was too anxious to eat.

His mother told me he asked her hourly if she was going to die. They were trapped in an anxious prison of his fear of death. Salah said he thought he would die because he and Jeremy's dad coincidentally had the same birthday. The family was in a death anxiety loop and they couldn't see a way out.

When Salah came to see me, we worked to separate the terrible tragedy of his friend's father's death from his own life story. He needed to grieve for this attachment figure he had grown up with. He needed clear reassurance that his parents were healthy. He needed time to be a child again and he needed to feel physically safe so his mind could slow down and give him space to recover.

From the beginning of this book, I have illustrated that at the base of every child's anxiety, deep down is the fear of death. In this chapter, the link between anxiety and death is much more obvious. You can see clearly exactly what frightens and worries your child.

Proximity to death – whether it's that of a family member, person in our wider sphere or even a character dying in a TV programme – makes all of us consider and fear it. It is an evolutionary safety response to make sure that if a person has been killed because they were bitten by a snake or electrocuted, we take suitable precautions to ensure the same thing doesn't happen to us.

Even adult brains, when faced with death, find it very hard to stay calm, assess likelihood and to understand that some diseases are contagious and some are not.

For children, there is an additional fear attached to death. If our parents or an important person in our life dies, we might not get what we need, such as care, food, medical attention and love. Therefore, we might die too – from neglect rather than illness.

Our bodies are working so hard to protect us from either outcome – that is, catching the disease or being neglected if our parents die – that the cortisol coursing through us causes an all-encompassing panic.

Signs that a child may be having death anxiety include:

- Constantly talking about death or dying.
- A sudden increased awareness of safety or danger.
- Sleep changes including nightmares and struggles to relax at bedtime.
- Increased separation anxiety.
- Somatic pain like headaches and stomach aches with no obvious cause.
- Avoiding things that bring up their fear of death, e.g. not wanting to go in cars after someone has had an accident.
- Not wanting to do things for themselves, like getting dressed, to make sure an adult comes to help so they can prove to themselves they are being looked after.
- Changes in mood or behaviour.
- Becoming more withdrawn, irritable, or aggressive.
- A noticeable change in their play, such as acting out scenarios involving death or loss.

- Talking about the world in a more existential way, e.g. wanting to discuss the afterlife or the meaning of life.

You can take action to help manage death anxiety, both when navigating a surprising death and before and after an expected death that there is time to prepare for.

In the case of a surprising death, children will have to contend with the shock as well as the fear that death brings. The aim is to give children a timetable of events that makes sense to them and helps them understand how rare and irregular this is.

In the case of an expected death, children have time to ruminate and panic and make up misconceptions to try and protect themselves from death. The hope is we can separate this death from the misunderstandings and help children prepare to celebrate life and grieve.

My feeling is that children can withstand anything if they know they will be looked after and that as little as possible is going to change.

In the face of death, you are trying to establish these ideas as facts for your child:

- You are safe.
- You will be looked after.
- Your life is going to continue as similarly as possible.
- We can survive this.

To make sense of death and explain mortality, we usually say two things: 'Old people die' and 'Ill people die'. So, we inadvertently teach children that death happens mainly to old, ill people. We are conditioned to use phrases like: 'He could finally stop fighting' and 'It would have been a relief at the end'. These do not prepare us for most of the deaths we experience, as no one we know ever seems old enough or ill enough to die.

Our brains have an understanding of death called *mortality salience*. It gives us the ability to ignore how close we are to death most of the time. Most of the time, we can ignore our mortality salience, as if we think too much about it we would be unlikely to leave the house; we'd be scared of passing cars, loud noises, all food . . . We would be consumed by both fear and sadness, as we would be engulfed by the proximity of death. If, however, we are shaken by a near-death experience, our mortality salience is rattled and we lose the shield or curtain that usually masks our awareness that death constantly hovers nearby.

Before death: where no one you know has died but your child is showing death anxiety

In the past few years, I have seen many children who have suddenly become extremely scared of death without losing a family member or close adult. Children absorb items on the news, overhear adult conversations and get told things by other children that can cause chaos in their heads. Children can pick up an awareness of a situation even if its context is less explicit. Children can see when their parents are scared, angry, upset or worried.

This mixture of misunderstood information and picking up on the atmosphere created by the adults in their circle can lead children to get a sense that something is terribly wrong even if it's just that you are feeling sad about an earthquake overseas.

Here's how you can help:

Identify the Misinformation

Ask questions to work out what they are thinking about:

- Did they hear something at school or on the news?
- Have they misunderstood a political situation?
- Is it a scary seasonal thing, like Halloween, or something they have seen on the internet that people are talking about?
- Is there an unwell teacher at school?

You can use the scripts from Chapter 3 if you need further support.

Give Concrete Ideas

Whatever issue comes up, think about how you can make it less frightening. If it is a horror movie, someone ill at school or a political conflict, consider the facts your child would need to understand to make it clear they are not under threat. Show them how far away the event was on a map; talk about the fictional nature of horror movies, which are purposely made up to frighten people. They are not real. Take the sting or heat out of stories other children talk about at school. Think about information that could be used factually to take the disturbing factor out of the situation.

Add Additional Physical Safety

When children's defences have been permeated by death-centric information, your job is to remind them how safe they are. You can do that by reminding them about how close we are, how lucky we are to live in a place where houses are safe. Run through the safety features of your home, sit with them a little longer at bedtime.

Give Opportunities to Calm the Body

When children have been overwhelmed by this fear of death, we need to help them relax into a feeling of safety. You can do this by adding an extra calming element when your child is at home. Add some yoga, calm music, lots of cuddles and family time. Be present and aim to slow everyone down and increase your presence and connection until you see your child's body relax.

Before death: when someone is terminally ill and you have time to prepare for this death

In the event that you know someone is unwell, but may die in a couple of months or years, it may be important to speak to the ill person and decide what they would like your child to know or not know. You can then take their wishes into account as you decide what you think is right for your family.

To help your child manage the anxiety that comes with this kind of news, your focus is to help your child know they will continue to live happily and safely no matter what. You may also wish to use this time to make memories and embed the ill person into your child's heart.

The aim is to protect your child from the possible impact of this death even if you do not feel the assurances you are giving them are strictly true. Your job is to be the fortress that keeps them feeling safe and looked after no matter what else is going on.

You will need to have a conversation with your child to start this process. For example, you might say: 'Hey bud, I have some things I need to talk to you about later. It's nothing to worry about, just something I think you should know about.'

The next step is to think of a quiet time to share the news. It could be on a walk in the park, at a café or in the living room before dinner or a family activity.

241

Give your child something crunchy to eat like cucumber, crisps or crackers to stimulate the vagus nerve – this reassures the body there is nothing dangerous going on. (They are safely grazing like an animal in a field.)

The aim overall is to give clear, understandable information, allow all their feelings to be acknowledged and accepted, and to make it clear that *you* are managing this new situation for them. At each stage of the conversation, aim to leave space for questions and feelings that come up for your child.

It might sound like this:

> Parent: So, I told you there was some new information I wanted to share with you. The news is a bit sad but it's nothing to worry about. Yesterday we found out that Uncle Steve is not very well and actually he has an illness that is not contagious but it means that he is going to die.
>
> *[Stop and breathe – regulate yourself and show your child that this news, while sad, is not too much to manage. You can cry and have your own feelings but aim to show your child that although you are upset, you are still capable of dealing with the situation. If you cannot share the information without crying uncontrollably, maybe wait a few more days or ask another close family member to share the news on your behalf.*
>
> *When talking about illnesses or accidents that have happened to others, the important thing for our children to understand*

is that the same thing is NOT LIKELY to happen to them. Explain that the illness isn't contagious or that they are highly unlikely to ever find themselves in the position that the other person was in.]

Parent: Uncle Steve is in hospital and the doctors and nurses are looking after him, but sadly his illness had spread to too many parts of him to fix. He is very ill now. He has an illness you cannot catch; none of us have it but we feel very sad for him that he has it and is now so unwell.

[Stop and breathe again – make space. Your child may ask a question, or want to cuddle or tell you something.]

Parent: Although this is very sad and we will miss Uncle Steve when he dies, we will say goodbye to him in our own way and then we will remember him so often it will be as if he is here with us. I know Uncle Steve usually takes you to gymnastics on a Friday and so Grandma will be doing that instead and we will still have our family dinners on Sundays where we can think about Uncle Steve and still be together as a family.

[You may feel as if the conversation has been sparse or emotionless. The point of it was to provide clear information and make sure there are no misconceptions in the original telling. There is always time to go back and talk about any part again or to sit and cry or shout together.]

Parent: Do you have any questions?

Dealing With Questions

You may at this point be asked questions about:

- The afterlife.
- Your death.
- Your child's death.
- Illnesses.
- Doctors' ability to save people.
- A logistical problem they are worrying about.
- Nothing – they may seem fine and skip off.

Whatever their reaction, your job is to try and answer their questions as clearly as possible.

For questions about:

The afterlife – Discuss with your partner or close family what you believe before this question comes up. Then explain what your family believes, leaving opportunities for questions.

Your death – Explain that you don't have that illness, that you are generally healthy and strong and that you plan to live for a very long time. If that is not enough, tell your child more about what you do to keep yourself healthy, and explain that as soon as you feel unwell you see a doctor and have experience of doctors helping you. If they are still worried, consider going for a health check at your GP or booking a one-off private appointment to reassure your child and tell them that's your plan.

Your child's death – Your child may ask if they are going to die and at that point you do not lie. You say, 'Eventually every-body dies but it is very unlikely that you will die soon. Do you know the average age people live to in the UK is eighty-one! That's the age most people live to, but lots live longer than that. You are X years old so that means you are likely to live for at least X more years! It's definitely not something you have to worry about today.'

Illnesses – If your child asks for more information about the illness your family member has or the accident they died in, make sure your response is age-appropriate. Sometimes chil-dren need a name of an illness to check it isn't something they have had before. Other times you do not need to give it a name, just say, 'It isn't something you can have at this age.' Or: 'It's very unlikely that you could ever get it.' Remind them it is OK to cuddle the ill person if they are not contagious.

Doctors' ability to save people – They may ask, 'But doctors are meant to fix people, why can't they fix Uncle Steve?' I would give fair but true information. You may also need to explain that certain very rare medical conditions are not cur-able. You can even share the idea that the fact that you know someone who had this illness means that you are even less likely to get it as it's so rare – look up the stats to help make your case.

Timelines – How long has he been ill? What treatment has he had before? Did he wait too long to see a doctor? Did he find out late? Did the accident happen for a surprising reason? Have your answers ready for all these types of questions.

Human error – Explain that although doctors go through extensive training and usually fix and save everyone, they are still human and can make mistakes. Try not to apportion blame, even if you are privately angry about some aspect of the treatment, as this could cause further fear and upset in your child.

A logistical problem they are wondering about – You may feel surprised and possibly a little disappointed when the thing your child asks after such sad news is something mundane and selfish, but we know that children will be trying to make sense of this news by comparing it to what they have known before. News like this is usually too big for most children to think of a suitable question. Answer their logistical issues honestly and let them know that if you don't have a plan, you will soon.

Children are trying to digest what you have said and asking questions can help you to be sure they haven't misunderstood. It is the misunderstandings that hold up children's grief processes and cause anxiety.

> **Firework idea**
>
> **When you both run out of things to say, end the conversation formally, but remind your child they can come to you and talk whenever they like.**

Preparation for the Death of a Close Family Member

- Give the child information you think they need to know and can understand.
- Explain the timeline as you know it.
- Ask children about the role that person plays in their life and what it might mean if they weren't there.
- Make space for all feelings and questions.
- Model healthy grief by going to therapy and calmly and kindly sharing your feelings.
- Organise therapeutic support for your child.
- Ask your child who they would like to know this news and ask if they or you should tell their teacher or their friends' parents.
- Make a list of things you know you want to do with that person and consider how you will make the time to actually get it done.
- Work on ways to spend time with that person while considering how to fill the gaps that will be left logistically.
- Start actively making memories, taking photos and asking the sick person questions about their life your child will want to know the answers to later – maybe do an interview recording.
- Ask the family member to make a playlist of their favourite songs.
- Make some art together.

- Arrange a weekend away with the unwell person and make that place their place so whenever you go there or talk about that place you can think of them.
- Think about and explain the funeral process to your child and work out which parts they will and won't attend.
- Organise a legacy project that will last after they pass away; this usually works best as a charity or community project.

You may never feel as if you have done enough to prepare your child for loss but you can aim for healthy grief and you can hope you and your child will be able to hold on to two important feelings at the same time: both the sadness of loss and the ability to celebrate and hold the feelings of love, happiness and connection from the past. If you have managed those things, you are doing a great job. You will be handling your own grief at the same time as managing your child's, even if your relationship with the deceased is different.

After death: a person has died in shocking circumstances

You might find the following script useful if you need to tell your child someone you know has died suddenly. Your aim is to minimise their anxiety as much as possible. First, set the scene by preparing your child for a conversation.

Parent: In a few minutes we are going to pop out for a walk / to a café / into the garden. I have something important but not worrying to tell you.

[Grab some crunchy snacks and water, to help calm the body and dilute cortisol levels as you talk. Arrive at your chosen location.]

Parent: I have had some very shocking and sad news and so I wanted to tell you so I could keep you in the loop and we could manage this together as a team. This news is / isn't about someone in your immediate family. Your teacher, Mrs Green, was on holiday for the half term and she has had an accident. She was _____ and something terrible happened and she was very badly injured. She then went to the hospital but _____. Sadly, although the doctors tried very hard, she died yesterday. I feel very upset about it as I am sure you do too.

What we know so far is _____ *[share logistical information]*. We know you liked Mrs Green very much and that this must be very confusing and sad news to receive. Do you have any questions?

Let them ask any questions, if the surprise has meant you aren't ready for the questions, just tell your child you will write down the question, think about it and get back to them. Then do so. Remember to make time to talk about it again.

Firework idea

You may find yourself talking a lot because this is such an awful and difficult conversation to have. Remember the silences will allow your child to feel whatever they are feeling. We do not want to rush them through this information or their feelings.

Parent: It is likely you will have lots of questions and feelings about this shocking news in the next few days and weeks and you can always come to me to talk, to cry, to just be together or to ask any questions that come up. I am also going to look into what support is available for you and if you want it at any point, it will be ready.

I think our talk is finished for now, what do you think you would like to do now?

You may feel as if the conversation has been sparse or emotionless. The point of this conversation was to provide clear information and make sure there are no misconceptions in the original telling. There is always time to go back and talk about any part again or to sit and cry or shout together.

Try to give physical contact here and a space for sadness, anger, confusion and anything else they may feel.

Firework idea

If you can, aim to tell your child at the beginning of a weekend so they have as much time at home in their safe place as possible before having to return to their normal schedule. Try to tell your child early in the day so they have longer to process their thoughts before bedtime.

After death: a person you knew was ill has died

You might find the following script useful if you need to tell your child someone you knew was ill has died. Your aim is to minimise anxiety as much as possible. Set the scene by finding a time when your child has nowhere to be afterwards, and a place to talk where they can be sad or show feelings without embarrassment. Make sure the conversation has a clear end point.

Let them know you are going to have to talk to them soon about something important but not worrying.

Parent: I have to tell you something sad and difficult, but I will help you manage this news so it doesn't have to be worrying. I know you knew that Grandpa had been unwell for a while and even though the doctors told us he might be alive for only a few months, he was actually with us for a whole year. This weekend, however, he began feeling unwell and as he was very ill with a slow-growing illness, they think that it finally spread too far because he died soon after he got to the hospital.

[Breathe deeply to regulate your own body, talk slowly and clearly. You are welcome to cry while you talk, but if you think you'll be so distressed it might make it hard for your child to understand the information, wait a little longer to share the news or ask someone else to help you.]

Parent: I think this will be very confusing and surprising news for you. I know we only saw Grandpa last Tuesday for dinner and he was telling stories and smiling. We have to remember he had been ill on the inside for a very long time with something you cannot catch. We can feel very sad he is gone, but also very lucky we spent so much time with him even though he was so ill.

[Take a deep breath, pause and see if your child asks you anything. It could be a good time to extend a hand or an arm for a cuddle.]

Parent: The next things that will happen are a funeral and _____. We have decided that for the funeral you will _____. I know how much you loved Grandpa and he loved you and that doesn't end even though he isn't here any more. Do you have any questions?

[Aim to answer questions that come up using the additional information from pages 244–6.]

Parent: I think we might have had enough of talking about this for now. It's a lot of new and sad information to take in. You can always come to me about any feelings you have or any questions you want to understand and I will always make time to be with you. All the feelings you are having now are allowed and correct and I am here for you no matter what. What would you like to do now?

Firework idea

Don't be surprised if your child returns to watching TV or playing after your conversation. We all need time to accommodate new information into our thought structures. Sometimes being passive while your brain sorts your thoughts out for you is more manageable when the information you have been given is so hard to understand.

How can you manage anxiety post-death for your child?

Weeks After

- Provide additional supports like time together, lifts to school, comforting meals and activities. Stay with them as they fall asleep if needed.

- Fill any emotional or logistical gaps left.
- Maintain their schedule as much as they can manage it.
- Support their sleep, quiet time and recovery.
- Look for therapeutic support if needed.
- Invite people over to talk about the deceased or go to a memorial for the deceased.
- Speak to your child's school and inform them your child might be sad or need extra leeway with deadlines.

Months After

- Maintain the connection with your child and set regular times to spend together.
- Help your child see that life continues after death; put some exciting events in the diary to look forward to and keep the most reliable events in the diary too, such as clubs they love, family dinners and school support.
- Find ways to celebrate the life of the deceased.
- Give opportunities for your child to talk about the deceased and how they miss them.
- Consider a charity project to commemorate them.
- Maintain therapy if needed.

Years After

- Help your child turn their grief and anxiety into happy remembrance by helping your child hold their relationship in mind.

- Have photos visible, talk positively when you can and, if applicable, show your child how they share positive traits with the deceased.
- Maintain your charity project.
- Help your child to assess how they have changed in the time since this death.
- Help them see how brave they have been and how safe they are now.

What support is available for children going through grief or fear of death?

- Grief counselling or therapy – this includes art therapy, play therapy and CBT. You can access this support through a grief charity, your school, the NHS or privately.
- Bereavement support groups for families, parents and children – these can be organised by charities, religious organisations and local councils.
- School-based support – this might include opportunities for counselling, social groups and additional accommodations like time out of class, more time for homework or delaying tests and exams.
- Support given by hospice care – this can include other more specific programmes for grieving families.
- Summer camps – look into special camps specifically for grieving children or siblings of ill children.
- Specific groups and activities – there are special groups for children who are facing specific types of bereavement,

e.g. survivors of accidents, children from military families or those who have lost a sibling.

- Community support – this might include events, groups and religious or spiritual guidance. The US-based Dougy Center or Child Bereavement UK offer such programmes.
- Online forums – there are many online communities dedicated to grief.
- Online resources – websites like Winston's Wish or Sesame Street's grief workshops offer tools and activities.

Firework idea

Another way to prepare young people for the death of an important person is to practise talking about death and even giving the news of a death when a famous person or pet dies. It won't make grieving a loved one easier, but it will show them life goes on after death, it makes talking about death less taboo and it gives you a chance to model healthy discussion for your family.

Books to help your child with death anxiety		
Children	**Teens**	**Adults**
The Invisible String by Patrice Karst	*What to Do When the News Scares You: A Kid's Guide to Understanding Current Events* by Jacqueline B. Toner	*Overcoming Loss* by Julia Sorensen
The Memory Box by Joanna Rowland		*A Child's Grief: Supporting a Child When Someone in their Family Has Died* by Di Stubbs, Julie Stokes and Katrina Alilovic
When Dinosaurs Die by Laurie Krasny Brown and Marc Brown	*Michael Rosen's Sad Book* by Michael Rosen	
Badger's Parting Gifts by Susan Varley	*Milo and the Restart Button* by Alan Silberberg	*Grief in Children: A Handbook for Adults* by Atle Dyregrov
Muddles, Puddles and Sunshine: Your Activity Book to Help When Someone Has Died by Diana Crossley and Kate Sheppard	*You Will Be Okay: Find Strength, Stay Hopeful and Get to Grips With Grief* by Julie Stokes	*Never Too Young to Know: Death in Children's Lives* by Phyllis Rolfe Silverman
The Garden of Hope by Isabel Otter and Katie Rewse	*Welcome to the Grief Club* by Janine Kwoh	
What Happens When a Loved One Dies by Dr Jillian Roberts	*The Million Pieces of Neena Gill* by Emma Smith-Barton	
Someday by Alison McGhee	*My Parent Has Cancer and It Really Sucks* by Marc Silver and Maya Silver	
What Does Dead Mean?: A Book for Young Children to Help Explain Death and Dying by Caroline Jay and Jenni Thomas	*Summer Bird Blue* by Akemi Dawn Bowman	
The Hare-Shaped Hole by John Dougherty & Thomas Docherty	*When a Friend Dies: A Book for Teens* by Marilyn E. Gootman	

When I'm Gone: A Picture Book About Grief by Marguerite McLaren and Hayley Wells *Mum's Jumper* by Jayde Perkin *Dear Star Baby* by Malcolm Newsome	*A Grieving Teen: A Guide for Teens and Friends* by Helen Fitzgerald	

Ten

Help! My Child is Anxious About Our Divorce and It's Giving Me Anxiety!

What are the very real fears hiding behind this anxiety?

- The fear everything you know is no longer true, making it harder to survive.
- The fear your life will never be the same again.
- The fear you will be different from other families.
- The fear you will never have the safety and security of two parents in one home again.
- The fear one of your parents is bad, incapable, unwell or too unhappy to care for you.
- The fear you cannot trust your parents again, as you trusted them to be together and now they are not.
- The fear there is now a Mum team and a Dad team, and it feels as if you can't be on both.

This chapter was written with the support of Talya Ressel. Talya is a clinical social worker psychotherapist born in South Africa. Talya used her experience helping children in schools manage divorce to become an internationally acclaimed speaker and writer on divorce and therapeutic family issues. She created Co Parenting Now, which has supported hundreds of families to set up their new lives post-divorce with their children's needs and mental health at the heart.

Why is divorce so anxiety-inducing for children?

Adults often underestimate the impact that divorce has on their offspring; children will experience the break-up of their parents' marriage like a bereavement. From their point of view, all that they know has ended and with it their sense of security. Even when they live in a home that is unsafe or full of conflict, that is what they are used to and children believe that is what their life will always be like. They know divorce will change their lives in a substantial and dramatic way.

Unlike a parental bereavement, there is no immediate assumption that children of divorce will miss school, enter therapy, or need additional help when it comes to sharing that information or experiencing the feeling of difference it brings. There is no specific charity, service or summer camp for children of divorce. They are often expected to continue to live and go to school without any extra support.

Obviously, children will adjust to this change over time, but it still causes a rupture or trauma that is very difficult to navigate and creates a raft of anxieties. At the same time, as long as you can contain your child's emotions, support them and show you can handle the changes in your lives, you will minimise the fallout and help them survive it better.

Shock can also cause major anxiety when the fighting or the conflict has been hidden, or the reasons the parents are divorcing have been concealed from the children because they are too complex for them to understand. The shock can make the greatest impact, so it's important that the surprise element is handled carefully.

In other cases, it's the continued conflict *after* the divorce that causes the most anxiety. Children can be caught in the middle and feel that there is no chance for peace or safety even when their parents are apart. It can make them feel that life is chaotic and scary.

Children can be played off between the two parents, be shamed for continuing to love one of their parents or find that arguments mean they have no reliable structure about where they will be or which parent they will see each week. Each child knows they are made equally by both parents and they can internalise shame if one is painted as a 'baddie'. Children may have a feeling of 'something's wrong with me', or 'I love Dad but Mum is saying bad things about Dad. Should I not like Dad?', or 'Am I being disloyal to my mum?' Divorce can bring up so many confusing and conflicting feelings.

In the face of divorce, we're trying to establish these ideas as facts for our children:

- You are safe.
- You will be looked after.
- You are still loved by both of your parents.

- Your life is going to continue as similarly as possible.
- We can survive this.

> **Firework idea**
>
> **If you have a bit of forewarning that you are likely to get divorced, see if you can set your child up with a therapist, a school mentor or a regular time to be with some other members of your family each week so that you have support structures in place for when the big changes occur.**

What is the best way to decrease anxiety when telling your child you are getting divorced?

Where possible, parents should aim to be together and on the same page when they tell their children. It's really helpful for the child to have a unified script from the parents with both telling the same story in the same way. The aim is to explain clearly but also provide reassurance to the child.

In an age-appropriate way, you are trying to make the new circumstances clear. Try saying: 'Mummy and Daddy have decided that we want to get divorced, which means we will not live together any more and we won't be married any more.'

Then begin to provide information and reassurance: 'Nothing is going to change about the way we both love you to the moon and back. I will always be your mummy. I will always be your daddy. We will always love you.'

Next, explain: 'What's changing is the romantic love. Sometimes, though grown-ups love and respect each other they are not "in love" with each other any more. This doesn't ever happen with parents and children. Parents' love for their children starts and never stops. It's not a two-way street; you don't have to earn my love. I love you because you are my child and I always will. A parent will always love you but romantic love between adults is different. Sometimes it changes and Mummy and Daddy are not in romantic love any more.'

You then set out the next steps as clearly as you can at such an early stage: 'We've decided that we need to live separately and Daddy is going to stay with Grandma for the next few weeks until we can make a better plan for where he will live. We will keep your activity schedule the same and we will both pick you up and take you to school on different days.'

Finally, you make space for questions. If you're both on the same page you will be able to think of answers that feel fair to both of you. Then your child can get clear united answers, which will make the prospect feel less scary.

Unfortunately, this united approach doesn't often happen because the parents' own emotions understandably are running high and it's hard to put your children first when you are wounded and in pain yourself. Explain to your partner how even if you aren't seeing eye to eye, setting the new, safe system up for your kids should be your priority.

If it's not possible to be on the same page, give a short answer or tell your child you'll get back to them once you have had a chance to think about it. Then remember to get back to them!

Firework idea

If you are divorcing under difficult circumstances, ask your co-parent for a truce when it comes to talking about your child. Say you will make your best effort to speak to them respectfully and kindly when it is about the school, home or social life of your child. Try to keep all other topics off the table to maintain your truce.

How do you then manage your child's expectations of the change?

Once you have had the initial conversation, you then need to reassure the child about the practicalities of the change in your circumstances. You are aiming to give as much information as possible. My feeling is that children can survive anything if they feel the adults have a solid plan and their daily lives are kept on an even keel and don't alter drastically.

You need to explain what a new week after your separation is going to look like. Children need concrete examples. You must try to give them a schedule as soon as possible and tell them that the schedule can change, but for the next two months or till the next school holiday, you have agreed with your co-parent you will try to stick to it to show that you are a team and that you can manage in this new structure.

When you have decided on the weekly plan, draw it up and print it out. Put it on your fridge. Put it on your co-parent's fridge. Then help your child think through what they will need to feel comfortable on the nights spent with their other parent. Ask questions calmly, such as: 'Would you like to take some things to your other home?' Then talk through the schedule: 'You'll still be going to football and you'll still be going to gymnastics. I am picking you up on Tuesdays, Wednesdays and Fridays and Mum will be doing the other days.'

Firework idea

Set a fair expectation with your co-parent – your child will do whatever is on the timetable during your days. The parent must arrive on time with the right items for those activities. Children will be returned to the other parent clean, well-rested and fed. Parents will not unfairly pry about the lives or homes of the other parent.

Break it down into practical situations. Your children might need a mini timetable that they keep in their school bag to see who's picking them up or where they're sleeping that night to minimise uncertainty as much as possible.

You can also ask them, 'Do you want me to tell your teacher? Do you want me to tell your friends so that you don't have to speak about it? Or do you want to tell them?'

You are aiming to give them some power and a lot of information to be able to make the best decisions as they get used to this new life.

> **Firework idea**
>
> **If you have big events coming up like birthdays or religious holidays, try to get plans in place early. Let your child know who they will be with on the day and what the other parent will do to celebrate on the next day they are together. Ask your child if they are happy with the plan and, if possible, give them a chance to say they'd like it to be the other way around. Talking about things well in advance gives all parties an opportunity to be happy with the plan and allows everyone to continue celebrating the good times.**

Dealing with resistance to the new routine

If children are having a difficult time with a transition – for example, they don't want to go to one parent's house – how do you help them get through it, particularly if that parent is a safe and previously well-regarded parent?

First, you want to acknowledge to yourself that they're going to have all these different feelings and it's a normal reaction to resist change. You need to handle this carefully.

Establish that the other parent's home is a safe environment and there's no tangible reason they don't want to go except that they feel conflicted about the divorce.

It can be useful to talk about or blame 'the schedule' rather than the co-parent. Say, 'I know you don't want to go tonight, but the schedule is that tonight you are at Mum's house and then you'll come back here tomorrow after school.'

Try to enforce what the schedule says in an age-appropriate way. You may have to negotiate as they get older and give them more chances to choose where they go, but for now, sticking to the schedule can stop children playing parents off against each other and shows that both parents are committed to the new family plan. It helps restore a feeling of consistency for the child even if they think they don't like it. It also helps children get used to it more quickly as they keep doing the same thing each week. Use the schedule as a third party or boss you can blame but still follow.

It's also a good idea to have a set time to call your child on the days they are with the other parent. Set a reminder to call them at 6 p.m. on non-parenting days. Even if they are busy and don't want to chat with you, you are maintaining your connection and showing that you are thinking about them when you are apart.

Help your co-parent do the same. Try to call at least an hour before bedtime so they can have time to settle and relax with the other parent before they go to bed.

Dealing with different rules in your co-parent's house

You may find that things are done differently at the other home: screen-time rules or junk food availability, for example. How can you manage your own anxiety about what goes on in the other house?

One of the most difficult parts of a divorce is the realisation that the amount of time you will spend with your children will change. In some cases, you may be with your children less and that can be even harder if you are worried about what they are doing in their other home. Ideally, parents should try their best to reach an agreement about what's best for their children. The most important thing is that whatever happens in the other home, it is a *safe environment*.

Parents should try to be consistent. It is tempting to be a 'Disney Dad' or 'More is More Mum' to try to keep your children happy and on your side, but being a 'yes parent' gives children too much power and can make them feel out of control at what is already an unsettling time.

You are aiming to keep things clear, calm and secure. Establishing a regular routine and boundaries in this new situation will directly counter the anxiety your child will feel and reassure them they and their all-consuming feelings can be contained.

The key is communication. The more you both talk, the more you will feel listened to and valued as the other parent for this family. Share information and communicate details, e.g. if they were ill, if they've been to the dentist or if they didn't fancy going to their chess club today. Talya says:

> I tell parents to set up a WhatsApp group for just sharing information about your child. For example, they have an extra rehearsal tomorrow, there were no socks in the PE bag or they had a falling-out with a friend. Even a quick message will help both parents do a better job when they are in charge and give them an opportunity to share problems inside that structure. This stops the need for children to be go-betweens or feel pressure to fill in both parents when they are struggling.
>
> I also suggest, at least for the first year or so, meeting with a professional mediator or third party for a check-in and a rejig of the schedule every three months. A professional can help you address the fact that your child is coming back tired and help your co-parent see what is best for the child without judgement.
>
> I think parents should know that moving between two homes actively builds resilience and life skills as children learn to manage different people, rules and

expectations. It'll be hard for all of you but with the aim of supporting your child as a priority, you can know you're doing all you can.

A divorce lawyer I've worked with for years said, 'The best divorces are when both parties feel as if they have lost.' This is because if both co-parents feel they have had to compromise, they are keen to be fair to each other and try harder to work together.

How to deal with your negative emotions towards your co-parent

If your co-parent has done something to upset or hurt you, how can you work to support your child to have a good relationship with that parent even though you are annoyed with them? Talya's advice is clear:

> It's important to separate the person from the parent. Sometimes someone can be a really sh*tty partner, but still be a good parent.

> You want your child to have the best possible impression of their other parent. I know it's asking a lot from a person in pain, but ultimately it benefits you and your children if you can help them have full relationships with both parents.

Discuss your hurt or anger with your friends or family, go to therapy and work to find a way to help your child preserve the best image of their other parent you can create. When a child has a good relationship with both parents, it sets them up to maximise their sense of safety and security.

You don't want your children to have to manage the changes of divorce while also feeling abandoned, separated or rejected, or that they are missing out on having good, kind parents who will look after them. Talya continues:

> Parents will often say, 'Shouldn't I tell my child the truth about what their other parent has done?' I would say 'NO!' It's likely what they have done is not age-appropriate and could cause more confusion, anxiety and fear. If it's not affecting their parenting, what I have come to find is that as children grow up, they start to see for themselves what their other parent is like. And as painful as that is, it's beneficial that they see it for themselves rather than the other parent pointing it out. The risk is they might blame you for warping their opinion of their other parent and spoiling their relationship.

> Don't lie, but wait until your child notices things about their other parent on their own *and* is old enough to understand what happened in a thoughtful way before you actively break down the image they have of their other, previously considered safe, parent.

Navigating new relationships

Anxiety can erupt when one or both parents begin new relationships. What is the best way to navigate this to reduce anxiety?

We know that for children of divorce, even adult children, a new partner for either parent brings on a primal grief. This is because, even though life has moved on, children often still think there might be a chance their parents could get back together until the point at which they are matched up with someone else. Children often have to grieve all over again for their hope for reunion and have no choice but to understand there's no going back. This can be very painful.

For the co-parent, it can also be a horrible feeling. Clear communication between co-parents helps. Establish clear boundaries about your child's exposure to you or your ex-partner's new love interest.

Talya says: 'Your ex should ask you and you should ask them first before you introduce your new love interest to your child. You don't need their permission to date or have a new person in your life but you do need to let them know. You'll let them know about this person because you respect them and don't want your child telling the other parent about this new partner. It's not their job to share adult information. I encourage talking with children or co-parents only when it's a significant relationship.'

When it comes to telling your child that you have met some-one else, Talya recommends waiting until you're sure it's a significant relationship before you break the news:

> If you see that there's longevity in this relationship, in the sense that you think a person is going to be in your life for the near future, i.e. the next year or six months minimum, you can begin to think about talking about it. You want to know there's an established base for a relationship. It's confusing for children if new partners come and go. So, in an ideal situation, I would start by saying to your child and your co-parent, 'I think that I'm going to go on some dates,' or 'I'm going to start meeting new people.'
>
> Then you can mention, 'I'm going for coffee with someone I met recently.' You are aiming to start dropping little pebbles of information that your children can understand are about a romantic relationship, but don't make anything concrete until you are sure. Then you can say a little later on, 'I actually am spending more time with this one friend.' You are aiming to give your child time to acclimatise to each stage before you rush to the next. You are also trying to see if this new possible partner is able to understand your relationship with your child and respect it and you at the same time.

If your co-parent has also had a slow drip feed of information, when you do ask them if your new partner might be able to meet your child, they won't be surprised and that might lead to an easier transition for everyone. Taking your time will also help you know if this prospective partner understands that your children come first – for example, they have shown they understand when you're busy and are kind about it. They need to grasp that single parents come as package deals with their kids. They are dating you *and* your children even if they haven't met them yet.

It's important for parents to find new relationships and have emotional nourishment and fun. Single parents are people too and deserve to step out of the chaos and enjoy themselves. When new relationships are managed slowly and transparently in an age-appropriate and respectful way to all parties, they can progress well and benefit everyone.

The key is to look at and listen to your own children. If you're dating somebody with their own kids, they might introduce you to their children before you feel comfortable doing the same with yours. You've got to do what's right for yours, especially while they are already processing such a big change.

What additional help is available for children going through divorce?

Talya says: 'I encourage parents to tell their child's school what's going on so that there are additional eyes on the child when they are out of the home and more support if they might be acting out at school.'

Also, if there's a school counsellor, it's helpful to have that space for your child to process their feelings in school and during the established timetable. It makes it easier, as children don't have to be picked up or dropped off by anyone. Therapy in school is different from private therapy. It's the school's job to organise consent and it may be able to happen regardless of the stage the parents have reached in their divorce proceedings. Private therapy, by contrast, needs clear consent from both parents and may not be an option depending on the current stage of the legal process that the family is going through.

Ask your school early on about in-school therapy so they can put you on a waiting list or make a plan for your child.

If therapy is not available, you can also find a parenting support practitioner or parenting expert to talk through plans without starting weekly therapy. It can help parents navigate the natural process of grieving and adjusting to their new life. After all, it is important for you to feel supported too, given the change is just as hard for adults as it is for children.

Family therapy versus individual therapy

You might think that family therapy is no longer an option for you after a divorce, but it's still worth considering. Talya says:

So, that's a thing with a divorce. You will always be a family and the best outcome for the child is that if you think forward in time, you will be sitting together at the child's wedding or at the birth of their child because that's what's going to be best for the child and what you'll want the most.

Even though you and your co-parent are not involved in a romantic relationship any more, you do want to try to foster some sort of new relationship. That's why family therapy can be helpful and it doesn't mean couples therapy. It's not for repairing your lost romantic relationship, but it does necessitate working together to be the best parenting team you can be. Sometimes I work with the parents separately but it's still under the banner or umbrella of family therapy because it's about creating a system that works as well as it can for *that* family.

Individual therapy gives children a space to be able to talk about the divorce and their life around the divorce without feeling as if they are declaring allegiance to one parent. It will give them a feeling of freedom to know that they won't upset the adult by talking about this difficult time. It usually takes place once a week. But remember, although regular time with an interested and qualified person can be useful, if the family system is still chaotic, there will only be limited change without a full system of support.

Other sources of support

Other support for children:

- Art therapy.
- Play therapy.
- CBT (see page 41).
- Websites: Voices in the Middle, Young Minds, Childline.

Other support for parents:

- DivorceCare – offers weekly support meetings.
- Co Parenting Now – run by Talya Ressel.
- Restored Lives runs courses and provides support for adults and children.
- Citizens Advice and Advice Now can provide legal advice and information to those going through divorce.
- Family Action runs a Separated Parents Information Programme that helps parents get the information and support they need to get through divorce.
- Parenting Apart Programme.
- Gingerbread organises support for single parents.
- Divorce Recovery Workshop.

Books to help your child with divorce anxiety		
Children	**Teens**	**Adults**
Where Did You Go Today? by Jenny Duke *Everything Changes* by Clare Helen Welsh *Roots of Love* by Sarah Asuquo *Two Places to Call Home* by Phil Earle *Two Homes* by Claire Masurel *Dinosaurs Divorce* by Laurie Krasny Brown and Marc Brown *My Family's Changing* by Pat Thomas *The Kids' Book of Family Changes: Understanding Divorce and Separation and Managing Feelings* by Catherine Stephenson *Two of Everything* by Babette Cole *Was it the Chocolate Pudding? A Story for Little Kids About Divorce* by Sandra Levins	*The Deepest Breath* by Meg Grehan *Dad's Girlfriend and Other Anxieties* by Kellye Crocker *What in the World Do You Do When Your Parents Divorce? A Survival Guide for Kids* by Kent Winchester and Roberta Beyer *To Night Owl from Dogfish* by Meg Wolitzer and Holly Goldberg Sloan *I, Cosmo* by Carlie Sorosiak *Step by Wicked Step* by Anne Fine *Divorce is Not the End of the World: Zoe & Evan's Coping Guide for Kids* by Zoe Stern and Evan Stern	*Talking to Children About Divorce: A Parent's Guide to Healthy Communication at Each Stage of Divorce* by Jean McBride *Shared Care or Divided Lives: What's Best for Children When Parents Separate* by Phil Watts *The Truth about Children and Divorce: Dealing with the Emotions so You and Your Children Can Thrive* by Robert E. Emery *Co-Parenting 101: Helping Your Kids Thrive in Two Households After Divorce* by Deesha Philyaw and Michael D. Thomas

Eleven

Help! My Child's Phobia is Giving Me Anxiety!

Miles was a happy, well-loved and liked eight-year-old. Near the end of Year 4, he went on a school trip. He had been feeling a little under the weather, but really wanted to try the high ropes activity that all his friends had been talking about for weeks. The journey was long and Miles began to feel very unwell. His teachers moved him to the front of the bus and looked after him, but forty minutes later he began being very sick. They pulled the coach over and he was sick many more times. In fact, he was sick so hard he burst a blood vessel in his eye and nearly passed out. Although he was well looked after, was quickly picked up by his dad and got better a few days later, he began to panic he would be sick again. He had developed emetophobia – the fear of vomiting.

This fear soon started to grow. Miles began to panic about car journeys, different kinds of food, catching germs and not being able to wash his hands. His fear stopped him enjoying his life and so his parents brought him to see me. Together we worked to restore his feeling of safety; we came up with logistical back-up plans for scary events, he spoke with a family friend who was a doctor about the rarity of dying from being sick and he learned how to look after his health without needing to panic. After a few months, he found his way back to being a happy little boy.

When does a worry become a fear or a phobia?

Daily **worries** are a normal and important part of being alive. We worry for all sorts of reasons – such as not having enough information about something, when we are trying something new and most importantly when we are sizing up potential threats and doing our best to keep ourselves safe in a situation.

A **fear** is usually triggered by a specific scary stimulus. Your child may have been scared by a character in a TV programme or a dog in the park. Maybe someone told them people eat spiders while they sleep and it freaked them out.

Phobias can also form because a child is feeling fearful, separated from their regular safety structures or out of control. To manage those feelings, they project their fear onto an object or a situation. This gives undue importance and power to something that would otherwise be trivial and unimportant. So, for example, your child might be sad and overwhelmed in bed at night because they are stressed about friendships at school, but their body cannot express the cause of their anxiety so they tell you they are terrified of the dark.

The important thing to remember is that phobias can be managed with support, compassion and sensible ideas.

When a child has a phobia, you may see:

- Avoidance of the thing they are scared of and everything connected to it.
- Irrational or excessive fear relating to that thing.
- Rituals being set up around those things to make them more manageable.
- Panic attacks.
- Either making a point not to talk about their fear or talking about it incessantly.
- Hypervigilance.

What are the first steps to fight fears and phobias?

The number one step I recommend is to *sort your fears*. Decide whether the fear presented is POSSIBLE or IMPOSSIBLE and then, if they are possible, are they RATIONAL/PROBABLE or IRRATIONAL/IMPROBABLE?

Possible	Impossible
Being left out at school	Ghosts
Being sick on a car journey	Being left at school forever
A parent getting ill or dying	Monsters
Being bitten by a dog	Loud noises like fireworks hurting you
Failing an exam	

Going to the dentist or doctor	The dark at home being dangerous
Climate change	Earthquakes in the UK
Balloons popping	Villains from films
Putting your hand in a waste disposal	Killer spiders in the UK
Getting stuck in lifts	
Injections	
Heights	
Thunderstorms	
Flying	
Blood	
Falling asleep	

Dealing with impossible fears

If the fear is impossible (and irrational), loudly and clearly declare that what they are scared of is *IMPOSSIBLE!*

As soon as it comes up that your child is scared of something impossible – e.g. snakes crawling through your pipes and ending up in the bath or toilet – tell your child, 'I know you saw that in a book/heard it from a friend/saw it on TV but that was *made up*. It never happens in this country. We don't have deadly snakes here and our pipes are specially designed to make sure animals and creatures can't enter them.' If you've been going along with this fear for a while by checking the bath or toilet for snakes, your behaviour may have confirmed your child's fears are rational, so change your approach conclusively. Tell your child your comprehensive research confirms their irrational worries will not occur. **Debunk** their fear.

Then start these next steps:

Use Your Experience

Use your age and experience to make it clear to your child that what they are fearful of will *not* happen. Say:

- 'That creature doesn't exist.'
- 'That does happen but not in this country.'
- 'That's just something to add excitement to books and films.'
- 'Never in my whole life, and that's thirty-seven years of being on this planet, have I ever heard or seen that happen to anyone.'

Make it very clear that you don't think that is a real thing or it wouldn't be a problem where you live.

Give Facts

Now explain *why* you think that. Aim to supply at least two different reasons why their fear has no basis in fact or wouldn't be a problem where you are.

- Show them on a map how far they are from the problem.
- Explain that with all the advances in technology and photography, we would have a picture by now of the creature if it existed and they would have its skeleton in the Natural History Museum.
- Tell them your house is always safe so just because the light is off or there is a loud noise, that doesn't change the fact that Mummy and Daddy are close by.
- Writers like to put things that you haven't seen before in books to make them interesting, but it doesn't mean they are true.

Help Them 'Talk to Their Brain'

When they begin to feel fearful, remind them of the facts and reasons their fear cannot and will not come true. Tell them to talk to their brain and tell it that this isn't frightening because it's not true.

Say, 'Oh! I can see your brain is telling you this is scary, but you know this isn't real/isn't going to happen. Now you can be in charge and tell your brain, "Hey brain" [ask them to repeat what you are saying] "You are telling me something is real but I know it isn't." Or "I'm safe and that isn't true." Or "Please calm down and listen to me!"'

This kind of speech can work in other moments of panic too.

BE AVAILABLE AND PRESENT

Even though you are working towards showing your child that this is not a logical stimulus for fear because it isn't real or dangerous, their brain still might think it is. They may need more connection with you while the information moves from scary to non-threatening in their brain. Our children may need a little patience, kindness and additional care as they work through their original anxiety and panic.

Cuddle more at bedtime, be close by when you can and realise this fear may take time to fully go away.

Talk About It as Many Times as Needed

I find that children under ten will need to talk about fears and getting rid of them lots of times before they can let them go. Children under five or with low speech may need a short-hand way to talk about their fear and may need to say it lots of times before they will allow it to dislodge and move on without it. Take a deep breath, streamline the conversation and know that in a few weeks there will be something else to talk about!

Don't Negotiate With Monsters!

I see lovely online pictures of beautiful handmade 'Monster Repellent' bottles or families writing letters from the Big Bad Wolf saying he has moved away. Although I can see why parents would want to use these whimsical methods to help their children's fears, it can be much more confusing and unsettling in the long run.

If we make monster spray, that means there *are* monsters. If I get a letter from the Big Bad Wolf, that means it exists and it could move back to where I live and eat me at any time.

Appeasing the fear can minimise it slightly, but it doesn't help our children differentiate and train their brains to identify what a real threat is. We know our children have a radar for threat that is working well – after all, the Big Bad Wolf or monsters are designed to trigger our alerts; they are bad characters or different from the norm – so it's important that they learn over time which threats require their full energy and which are designed to give a little bit of temporary excitement (in films, for example) but don't need to come home with them.

Dealing with possible fears

If the fear is possible – i.e. it *could* happen – start by sorting it into how rational or irrational it is and, from there, how likely or unlikely it is.

Rational	Irrational
Being left out at school	Balloons popping
Being sick on a car journey	Thunderstorms

A parent getting ill or dying	Blood
Being bitten by a dog	Falling asleep
Failing an exam	
Going to the dentist or doctor	
Climate change	
Putting your hand in a waste disposal	
Getting stuck in lifts	
Injections	
Heights	
Flying	

Likely	Unlikely
Being left out at school	A parent getting ill or dying
Being sick on a car journey	Being bitten by a dog
Failing an exam	Putting your hand in a waste disposal
Going to the dentist or doctor	Getting stuck in lifts
Climate change	Blood
Injections	Thunderstorms
Heights	
Flying	
Balloons popping	
Falling asleep	

By sorting the fears, we can decide what our position will be, and we can increase our child's feeling of security by using its descriptor to help us identify the best way to tackle their concerns.

- **Rational:** Focus on an empathetic approach – i.e. 'you are right to feel this way, it is scary' – then come up with a plan than provides clear information and support. For example, say your child is scared of going to the dentist because it might hurt. Tell them they are right, it may hurt, so you will make a plan with the dentist to minimise the pain.

- **Irrational:** Similar to how we focused on the impossible nature of monsters with their irrational fears, we want to show our children the reasons why what they believe is illogical and not based on fact. We should also aim to show them over time in small steps that their fear is unsubstantiated. For example, if your child was scared of balloons and loud noises, you could explain that even when balloons pop, they are generally safe. Then over time you would expose your child slowly and kindly to balloons, first a deflated balloon, then a partially inflated balloon and so on, until they are able to be near a balloon without support.

- **Likely:** Likely fears need plans that clearly mitigate their real-life impact. If your child is scared of dogs and you live by a park, they are likely to run into the source of their fear regularly, leading to increased panic and hypervigilance. You need to make a plan with enough layers of security so that your child would be able to trust you to support them and relieve their hypervigilance. For example, you might say, 'When we go to the park, we will hold hands or I will carry you until we are in the gated playground. If a dog comes towards us I will loudly say, "Please move your dog away from us as we do not like dogs."' Then ask your child if that feels like enough support; do they have any other ideas?

- **Unlikely:** Unlikely fears are based on fact but they are rare or only likely to happen under certain circumstances. If, for example, your child is scared you will get very ill, which is possible but unlikely, you should focus on giving your child facts to support their understanding that worrying about your possible ill health now is a waste of their energy and brain space. You can tell them that they can trust you to keep them informed and aware of any changes in the likelihood of it happening or the need to worry.

If it's a **situation-based fear**, like a fear of wasps, you can support your child with a clear plan whenever they have to be in a place with wasps. You might say, 'I will be the wasp monitor and if they keep coming to our table I will move us all inside.' In addition, when you are not near the source of the fear, you could remind your child that most people are not allergic to wasp stings and, although a sting would hurt, the pain finishes in around an hour and then you make a full recovery. Ask people who have been stung by wasps about it. Get yourself some information and pass it on kindly and safely.

How do I help my child rise above their fears?

Validate Fears

Show and explain that you understand why they are anxious, that the thing they're concerned about can be a bit worrying. Listen to what they say about their fear. Try to work out which part is making it stick. Is it how they found out about this thing? Is it people continuing to talk about it? Is it something for adults that they shouldn't have been exposed to? Is it something most kids wouldn't mind, but there has been a misunderstanding about something?

Worst-Case Scenario

If you think your child would benefit from talking about it in greater detail, maybe a few days after the first introduction of this new fear, ask them: 'I can see you are still worried about X. What do you think is the worst thing that could happen with that?' Follow it up with 'And then what would happen?'

For example, your child might say, 'I'm scared of going to the dentist.'

> Parent: What do you think is the worst thing that could happen at the dentist?
>
> Child: The dentist could hurt me by putting those sharp things in my mouth.

Parent: Wow, that does sound scary. And then what would happen?

Child: She could cut my mouth and it would bleed like it did last time and it could be really bad.

This child is identifying the link between pain, blood and death and it's making going to the dentist much scarier and anxiety-inducing.

Identify All the Misconceptions

Now you know what your child's negative assumptions are, you can work out where their logic has gone wrong and what their misconceptions are. In this case:

- It always hurts at the dentist and nothing can be done to make it less painful.
- I bled once at the dentist. What if it happens again and it bleeds too much?
- Do dentists know how to look after me?

Make a Plan and Give Facts

Using the misconceptions that have come up, find specific interventions to make each thing less overwhelming.

Pain – 'Well, I can hear that last time it was very painful, so how about when we go next time you can have some Calpol before we go? We can also talk to the dentist about whether she can use more numbing cream and ask if there are any other things she can recommend to make it less painful?'

Bleeding – 'If the bleeding is worrying you, we can ask the dentist if it's likely there will be blood in this check-up and whether the amount of blood last time was at all dangerous – because from what I remember, it was just a few spots on a tissue and that can happen while brushing at home.'

Dentist skill – 'I've chosen a really good dentist for children. I did my research and she is a registered dentist and extremely well trained. Maybe we could ask her about how she became a dentist and how often she looks after children?'

Give Child-safe Exit Strategies

Consider that sometimes just knowing that something will be over soon is enough to give children the strength to get through it. You might say: 'If you don't like it after thirty minutes, we can go home.' Or, 'If anything comes on the stage in the show that makes you feel worried, I will happily go outside with you and get something to eat instead.'

You can make prospects less daunting by setting a short time limit, asking they try something first, explaining the reason why you have to go and reminding them why that activity is important. Work to keep them as close to you as they need, help them stay calm or distract them with toys or conversation until they reach the end, and use the option to leave or stop if needed.

Consider Gradual Exposure

Gradual exposure is a method used in therapy to slowly acclimatise someone to the thing they are scared of. If your child has arachnophobia, for example, you might start by showing them a fun picture book with spiders in, then sitting on the grass in the park knowing there could be spiders around, then asking a trusted friend to flip a log in your garden and describe what's under there, eventually building up to the goal of visiting the spider room at the zoo.

Go slowly, building over time. Going too fast or making your child miss smaller steps could lead them to stop trusting your support and become even more fearful.

Other Ideas

- Teach grounding and breathing techniques – see the chapter on panic attacks or exam pressure (pages 383–6 and 174–8).
- Once you have made your plan to support your child, check in to see if it's working or if they have any other ideas or need a new plan. Help them gain and cement longer-term positivity by celebrating every small, brave step.
- Be the person in charge of this fear and show your child they can trust you to manage it for them.

- Make time to help their mind and body calm down – see Chapter 4, pages 102–105.
- Role-play about the fear.
- Use affirming language where possible. Say things like, 'You are doing so well; every time we go to the park I can see it's hard for you but your bravery is shining through.' Or 'Have you noticed you have now been to three different places with balloons and you got through it! It's very impressive, you should be so proud of yourself. You are building up so many examples for yourself of times you conquered your worries.'
- Consider that some activities or some parts of things are not imperative.

Firework idea

Enlist a feeling of teamwork. Five different studies run by Stanford University researchers show that even the most subtle feeling that you are on a team makes people more likely to be successful and productive in whatever task they are doing. Why not use this feeling of being on 'Team Overcome This Phobia' or 'Team Get Through This Hard Moment' to help take better steps to success and calmness?

How to not pass on your fears

Children learn by modelling their parents' behaviour. So how do you avoid them picking up on your fears if you have an unresolved phobia or anxiety?

- **Watch your language.** Aim to use positive language around your fears.
- **Model coping skills.** Say to your child, 'I do get scared but then I do my grounding exercises' (see pages 383–6).
- **Show your child your positive thought processes.** Show how you engage your rational brain to fight against your fears.
- **Say it out loud.** For example, 'I'm a little scared of lifts, but you don't have to be. I have so many experiences of safe lifts and you will have even more. It isn't your fear. You can follow your own instinct.'
- **Give your child space to make up their own mind.** If we hover around or look horrified when our child goes near the thing we are scared of, they will read your expression and internalise the fear. Teach safety skills then let them use them and help them make their own more positive associations.
- **Teach problem-solving strategies.** Problem-solving skills will come in useful in every area of a child's life. Ask your children to think through difficult situations regularly.

Firework idea

Ask your child what was difficult about their day and share something age-appropriate that was hard about yours. Then brainstorm different ways to solve or improve those tricky moments. If we do this regularly enough, our children will begin to employ this method of assessment and planning alone.

- **Think of ways to safely expose your child to your fear.** Ask a friend or family member to take your child in a lift, go with them for the injection or take them to the balloon shop. You don't have to pretend you are fine if you are not. There will be people who can help you and your child.
- **Think about finding some professional support.** If your fear is stopping you doing things daily, weekly or monthly and stops you from doing necessary parenting or working tasks, it may be time to see if personal therapy, CBT (see page 41), EMDR (see page 203) or hypnotherapy can help get it under control.

What support is available for children with fears or phobias?

- Child therapy/counselling
- CBT (see page 41)
- Hypnotherapy

- EMDR
- Dialectical Behaviour Therapy (DBT) – this is a kind of talking therapy that uses the practical approach seen in CBT. It's particularly useful for people who feel things very deeply as it helps them accept their emotions to become more present and in control
- EFT tapping (see pages 45–6)
- Coaching
- No Panic or Triumph Over Phobia (TOP UK) are charities that support those with phobias

Books to help your child with fears and phobias		
Children	**Teens**	**Adults**
Fraidyzoo by Thyra Heder	*Guts* by Raina Telgemeier	*Phobia Relief: From Fear to Freedom* by Kalliope Barlis
When Worry Takes Hold by Liz Haske	*Allergic to Girls, School, and Other Scary Things* by Lenore Look	*Play-Based Interventions for Childhood Anxieties, Fears, and Phobias* edited by Athena A. Drewes and Charles E. Schaefer
Me and My Fear by Francesca Sanna	*What to Do When the News Scares You: A Kid's Guide to Understanding Current Events* by Jacqueline B. Toner	
Franklin in the Dark by Paulette Bourgeois		
The Dark by Lemony Snicket		
Brave as a Mountain Lion by Ann Herbert Scott		
Thunder Cake by Patricia Polacco		

Twelve

Help! My Child's Food Anxiety is Giving Me Anxiety!

What are the very real fears hiding behind this anxiety?

- The fear you could die from choking.
- The fear food might make you unwell.
- The fear you might be unloved for being overweight.
- The fear your parent is very worried about you in a scary way.
- The fear food is chaotic and scary yet we need it to survive.

This chapter was written with the support of Lubna Dar, who is a counselling psychologist with more than twenty-five years' experience working in the NHS at the Maudsley Hospital in south London, providing health education for councils and for charities specialising in eating disorders.

Food anxiety is common in both parents and children. The reason is easy to understand. As soon as we become parents, we realise – on the most basic level – our primary job is to keep our baby alive. To make sure they survive and thrive, it's essential to keep them adequately fed. Naturally, we worry that we will somehow mess up this all-important task. We know that to keep our baby healthy, eating and sleeping are our primary concerns – and with baby sleep often being an impossible dream, many parents focus on eating to prove how well they are doing in their parenting.

Food anxiety in children frequently begins at around a year to eighteen months when babies are introduced to solids. You will notice your child's anxiety around food when they refuse to eat certain foods or show extreme reluctance. It will be difficult to work out why. You may never know if a lump in a certain food caused them to choke a little, or the taste of a particular food was unpleasant or too strong. What you will see is your child growing uneasy and tearful when a particular food is served.

What should you do about your child's food anxiety?

Take the heat out of the problem. Instead of anxiously saying, 'These are delicious pureed carrots. They are lovely. Have another mouthful for Mummy,' just remove the carrots from your child's sight and don't serve them again for a week. When you do, make them seem different from the last time. If they rejected pureed carrots, next time serve them raw or grated. If they reject carrots again, calmly take them away and wait a decent length of time before trying them again. Research shows that most children will take at least eight attempts to like a food they didn't immediately enjoy. The key is not to become fixated on particular foods and not to spoil your child's pleasure in the foods they do enjoy by show-ing anxiety and looking tense whenever they start to eat.

> **Firework idea**
>
> Look up a 'first 100 foods for babies' list online (there are several variations of these) – you'll see such a wide mix-ture of grains, proteins, fruit and vegetables. The idea is to use it to try to give your child as many different foods and textures before they are a year and a half. Put it on the wall in your kitchen and order a new food to prepare and then tick off every week. You can find a list free online like the one on the Once Upon a Farm Organics website. Start with the fruit and veg and, when it is age-appropriate, move on to the other sections. Make sure that on the day your child tries allergens, like peanut butter, you are with another adult in case of a reaction. These lists are designed for new eaters but can be used to diversify and gently challenge your child to try new foods.

What if my child only eats a few foods?

If your child refuses all foods except halved grapes, plain pasta and strawberry yoghurt, relax and serve them what they like. This won't go on forever. Every day put a little taste of some-thing else on their plate: a triangle of cheese, a slice of apple, a few grains of sweetcorn. Eat a varied diet yourself and have your meals alongside them so they can clearly see you enjoying a wide range of different foods. Tell them how scrumptious your piece of chicken or spaghetti Bolognese is. Offer them a taste. Keep joking and laughing. Make mealtimes fun. If all they end up eating is a few strands of pasta and a couple of spoonfuls of yoghurt, don't refer to it. When they are hungry, they will let you know they want something else to eat.

It's a good idea to give your child a supplementary children's vitamin, particularly in the winter months when there are bugs around (all children benefit from this, not just anxious eaters). Once you know your child will not go short of vital vitamins, your anxiety quotient will subside.

Firework idea

Consider going for a short walk after lunch or dinner each day. Going for a short walk can aid digestion, reduce sugar levels, make sleep more restful, increase heart health and be an easy routine to get into to increase dopamine, serotonin and endorphins. It also adds another relaxing opportunity to calm your child and spend time with them.

How do I take the anxiety out of eating?

The key thing here is to make eating fun:

- Have a picnic on the living-room floor.
- Involve your child in cooking and food preparation.

- Pick and use something fresh even if it's only basil from a plant on the windowsill or a couple of strawberries from the garden.
- Grow mustard and cress.
- Make the strangest sandwich your child can think of and taste it.
- Eat ice cream in the bath.
- See if you can eat a doughnut without licking your lips.
- Make fruit segments into funny faces.

Do anything and everything you can think of to make eating a fantastic experience. Your child can't be anxious if they are giggling. You can't be anxious when your child is laughing their head off.

Don't worry about mess

If you have food mess anxiety, do your best to plan ahead.

- Take your child's clothes off before meals and feed them in just a nappy.
- Put a big plastic sheet under the highchair or table to catch mess.
- Don't flinch if they put gravy in their hair or plunge their hands into the custard. It can all be washed off afterwards.

What you really want is a child who is happily immersed in eating. Sit near your child so there is no danger of their choking, but don't fixate on them while they eat. Listen to music, call a friend or just take a moment to eat and drink yourself. Allow them to make a mess, handle the food and get stuck in. That is what you are aiming for.

> **Firework idea**
>
> **Try to let children stay messy until the end of the meal unless the food is near their eyes or is uncomfortable for them. Wiping children in between spoonfuls of yoghurt can make them take their attention away from eating and create a negative sensory experience when you are trying to build new positive associations.**

What if my child under or overeats?

A child aged three or above who under or overeats may well be feeling anxious in other areas of life and showing their distress through avoiding or bingeing on food. Try to work out what might have happened to cause them to change their eating pattern.

- Has there been a change?
- Are they at a new school?
- Has a new baby been born?
- Has there been a death or divorce in the family?
- Is there anything else, even something seemingly minor – a glimpse of an unsuitable film, a guest in the house, a change in sleeping arrangements – that might have unbalanced them?

If you can't get to the root of the issue, but your child is definitely eating too much or too little, try to set eating structures that help your child eat in a more regulated way.

Serve the same amount of food for all young people in the house and leave the rest on the side in the kitchen. This gives children a chance to think about if they want or need more food.

Try to reduce the amount of screen-watching that occurs at the same time as eating. It can stop children listening to their bodies and make it harder for them to register when they are full up – or alternatively it can monopolise their attention so they avoid eating.

Set up a healthy and accessible food station in your kitchen that your child can go to with food that is filling and delicious but not processed or high in sugar. This may help your undereating child get into a routine of fuelling themselves and help your overeating child make more positive snacking choices and fill them up in a healthier way so they may eat less at other times.

If your worries are plaguing you, start by making an appointment to see your GP and ask for advice. They may refer you to a nutritionist, do further investigations around your child's health and diet or suggest your child have some therapeutic support.

What if my child is anxious about eating at school?

It is common for children to be anxious at the thought of eating in the unfamiliar environment of school. It can be intimidating to eat strange food in a strange place with strangers. If your child doesn't adjust to school food or eating their packed lunch in the school dining room within a couple of weeks, speak to the teacher and ask if you can pop along at lunchtime to talk them through it. Within a few weeks, most children get used to the routine of school dinners and many will happily eat foods they never touch at home just because their classmates are tucking in. For the first few weeks, be ready to feed your child more substantial meals at home because they simply might run out of time to eat all they need to be satisfied at school.

Other options to aid in-school food anxiety:

- Swap from school lunch to packed lunch or vice versa to see if that makes a difference.
- Ask if your child can eat facing away from the bustle of the lunch hall.
- Go through the school menu each day before school and help your child choose things they like from the list.
- Ask your school for more simple foods to be available every day like plain pasta or bread and butter.
- Ask the teacher to check if your child has a logistical issue with how they choose food, carry it across the room or find seating.
- Ask your child about the sensory experience in the school hall: is it loud, smelly, too overwhelming? How can you help to reduce the issue?

What if my child is anxious about social eating?

Your child may worry about eating at parties, during play dates or even at their grandparents' house. That is understandable. They don't know what they may be served and they are unaccustomed to the routine and environment. Try to talk them through it and prepare them in advance. Talk about the parties you went to as a child and the sorts of foods you enjoyed. You could reassure them you will phone the other parent before the play date and find out what they'll be serving for lunch. You can send them along with a lunchbox with a few of their favourite foods inside. The key here is to turn eating out into an adventure. They will not starve. They will not be poisoned. The food may not be exactly the same as you serve at home, but they have their little stash of snacks with them so they don't have to eat anything they really don't like the look of. On the other hand, tell them you think they would thoroughly enjoy at least having a tiny taste of the food served, just in case it turns out to be delicious.

How do I get the grandparents on board?

Explain your child's food anxiety to their grandparents. Make sure they understand your child is not being 'naughty' or 'picky'. It's entirely normal for children to like some foods more than others, exactly as adults do. Make it clear that you do not want your child to be made to eat anything they don't like and you certainly don't want them to be told off or punished for not 'clearing their plate'. On the other side of the coin, be very specific about your rules around sweets, chocolate, crisps and ice cream. This is your child. You have the right and responsibility to protect their teeth and make sure the calories they eat are doing them good. A little bit of spoiling is expected from grandparents, but you must establish clear boundaries.

What if I'm fearful my child's eating may be a sensory problem or related to neurodivergence?

If your child's food avoidance is linked to a sensory issue, you will most likely notice they have other sensory things that agitate them. They may notice noises, fabrics, tightness of clothes, heat and cold more than other children, how light it is, and the texture or colour of foods too. In this case I would aim to make them as sensorially comfortable as possible. Make the room quiet and calm when they eat, take their food notes seriously and try presenting the same food in other ways to change texture and consistency. Have safe foods or food that is always the same like crackers available so that they can find what they need without adding to their difficult experience at meal times.

Consider taking your child for a sensory assessment with an occupational therapist who will help you organise a sensory diet. A sensory diet is not primarily to do with food. It's a consideration of the different sensory experiences at school, home and the different places your child visits and it makes a plan for how to help dampen or increase the sensory input your child is receiving. This may be through the use of ear plugs, working or eating in a separate space or using proprioceptive intervention to calm the body (see pages 102–105).

Let's talk about ARFID and how it's treated

ARFID, or avoidant/restrictive food intake disorder, is an eating disorder or persistent disturbance in eating or feeding that leads to significant health issues, nutritional deficiencies, mental health problems and social isolation. Unlike other eating disorders, ARFID is not driven by body image concerns but by fear.

Children with ARFID may be fearful that food will make them ill or sick, that they could choke or be allergic to something they eat. This may be from a previous experience of this for themselves or people around them.

Children with ARFID are often small for their age, have lost a lot of weight or consistently miss height or weight milestones for their age. They may have an extremely restricted list of foods they can eat without fear. When tested, it can be seen that their very limited diet has caused deficiencies in their body. They may be regularly tired as they are not consuming food for the energy needed for each day. They can be dependent on supplements or nutritional aids like PediaSure. They may experience social issues as they may feel highly anxious about eating with other people or seeing others eat. They may have a notice-able lack of interest in eating or find the sensory experience of eating overwhelming or unbearable.

Treating ARFID is usually done by a team of professionals. A child may need nutritional rehabilitation, therapy, sensory integration through occupational therapy, medical monitoring, exposure therapy and maybe a support group.

Early identification and intervention are key to effectively managing ARFID and improving outcomes for those affected.

Help! I'm anxious about passing my own food issues on to my child!

If you are an under or overeater, constant dieter, food addict or simply use food to soothe your feelings, remember children copy their parents' behaviour. If you never sit down to eat, constantly talk about how fat you are, embark on different restrictive diets or reach for the biscuit tin when you are miserable, there's every chance your child will mirror your behaviour. We learn to keep many things private from our children. We don't talk to them about our sex lives or our financial problems. Do your best to keep your food issues far away from your children.

Sit down with them at mealtimes and eat anything you feel

comfortable with: a healthy mixed salad, grilled chicken, grilled fish, a pile of vegetables, soup, granary bread or any other food that sends out the right message. Food is delicious. Food is fuel. Food is pleasure. A varied diet of different foods is what this family needs and enjoys. If you have thoughts about how much or how little food you wish you had eaten or not eaten, do not express them in front of your child. Do your best not to hand your food issues over to your children. Of course, the very best way of all is to deal with and work through your food issues with a therapist or counsellor so they no longer have to be hidden from your children because you have managed to conquer them.

What if my child is approaching or passing puberty and seems to be developing an eating disorder?

If you think you see signs of anorexia or bulimia, your child may well be feeling out of control in other areas of life and seeking to establish extreme control over what they eat as a substitute. Many parents try their hardest to grapple with eating disorders by bribing their children to eat more or threatening them with punishment if they won't eat normal-sized meals. This method very rarely succeeds. Your child is struggling emotionally and showing it in their attitude and consumption of food. Seek professional help and advice. Anorexia and bulimia are complex conditions and the greatest favour you can do your family is to bring experts in to ease the problem at the earliest possible stage.

What support is available for children struggling with food anxiety?

NHS services:

- Visit your GP.
- Ask for a referral to the Child and Adolescent Mental Health Service (CAMHS).
- Ask to be referred to the NHS eating disorder services.
- For more complex cases, inpatient care can be organised.

Specialised eating disorder clinics:

- Private clinics such as the Priory Group and Orri – look up private eating disorder clinics in your area.
- The Maudsley Centre for Child and Adolescent Eating.

Therapeutic interventions:

- CBT (see page 41).
- Family-based therapy.
- Occupational therapy for children with sensory issues.

Dietary support:

- Dietitians with a specialism in working with children can help support with food integration, meal planning and food restrictions due to allergies.
- Feeding clinics are available in some hospitals to help children with more acute food issues to be helped to eat by a team of specialists including dietitians, OTs and therapists.

Charities:

- Beat is the UK's leading eating disorder charity. They run support groups, helplines and online resources for both children and their families.
- ARFID Awareness UK is a charity that provides resources, support and advocacy for those affected by ARFID.
- The National Autistic Society is for children with ARFID who are also on the autism spectrum. The NAS provides tailored advice and support.
- Young Minds – this charity focuses on children's mental health and offers resources, a helpline and online support for eating disorders.

School support:

- Many schools offer in-house counselling.
- Ask your school SENCO to organise Individualised Education Plans (IEPs) that help schools understand and support a child's food needs.

Parental support and education:

- Parent training and support groups are often run by charities and local councils.

Workshops and online resources:

- Organisations like Beat offer workshops online resources.

Emergency support:

- For crisis lines and local crisis teams, speak to your GP or dial 111.

Books to help your child with food anxiety		
Children	**Teens**	**Adults**
All Food Is Good Food by Molli Jackson Ehlert	*The Intuitive Eating Workbook for Teens: A Non-Diet, Body Positive Approach to Building a Healthy Relationship with Food* by Elyse Resch	*The Gentle Eating Book: The Easier, Calmer Approach to Feeding Your Child and Solving Common Eating Problems* by Sarah Ockwell-Smith
How We Eat by Shuli de la Fuente-Lau		
Welcome to Our Table: A Celebration of What Children Eat Everywhere by Laura Mucha and Ed Smith		*Helping Your Child with Extreme Picky Eating: A Step-by-Step Guide for Overcoming Selective Eating, Food Aversion, and Feeding Disorders* by Katja Rowell
Priya's Kitchen Adventures by Priya Krishna		
I Can Eat a Rainbow by Olena Rose		*ARFID: Avoidant Restrictive Food Intake Disorder: A Guide for Parents and Carers* by Rachel Bryant-Waugh
Hooray for Bread by Allan Ahlberg and Bruce Ingman		
Which Food Will You Choose? by Claire Potter and Ailie Busby		*How to Raise an Intuitive Eater: Raising the Next Generation with Food and Body Confidence* by Sumner Brooks and Amee Severson
Kew: Lift and Look Fruit and Vegetables by Tracy Cottingham		
Oliver's Fruit Salad by Vivian French		

Thirteen

Help! My Child's Body Anxiety is Giving Me Anxiety!

What are the very real fears hiding behind this anxiety?

- The fear there is something irregular or wrong with your body.
- The fear that you will stand out from others because of your appearance.
- The fear you might be unloved for being overweight/ underweight or looking different to others.
- The fear you will be socially ostracised for the way your body looks.
- The fear that to make yourself look a certain way you might have to put yourself in danger.

Studies show that children as young as three may begin to notice their bodies in a negative way. As children grow, their body awareness increases and negative attitudes towards their bodies peak in adolescence. It is deeply distressing for parents to hear their children use words like 'fat' or 'ugly' to describe their bodies from the age of five onwards.

If your child comes to you saying they feel unattractive, underweight, different or overweight, most parents respond instantly to their child's unhappiness by saying: 'NO! You are not fat/skinny/ugly. You are perfect!'

Instead, it is more helpful to your child to say:

- 'I'm so sorry to hear that, that must be a very difficult thing to feel.'
- 'How long have you felt that way?'
- 'What do you think started this feeling off?'
- 'Do you think it's useful to let things other people tell you dictate how you should feel? (Should Sarah be able to decide what people think? Is she an expert on bodies?)'
- 'How can we help you see how beautiful/strong/capable/just right you are for your age?'

List some of the wonderful things they can do with their body – run, jump, swim, dance, carry their sibling up the stairs, make a pancake – and show them all the positive attributes about their bodies you have noticed. Tell them you are always here to listen to any strange or upsetting feelings they may have about their bodies. You are very happy indeed to remind them how beautiful and strong they are.

What are the signs your child may have body anxiety?

Some children will say outright that they are unhappy or self-conscious about their body but other signs might be:

- Frequently checking out their appearance in mirrors.

- Seeming overly worried about what they wear.
- Changes in grooming techniques, particularly using make-up, straightening hair or wanting to spend lots of money on new clothes, to cover up something they think is unattractive or to look the same as others.
- Choosing not to engage socially because they cannot find the right clothes to wear or are worried about what other people may say about their appearance.
- Noticeable changes in eating to affect appearance – this includes dieting, missing meals or eating more than usual to gain weight or bulk up.
- Changing their style to very baggy or loose clothing to cover their body shape or a particular body part.
- Sleep disturbances or bad dreams.
- Increased anger or irritability when talking about their body or when they have to get dressed.
- Constantly talking about weight, size, body parts or appearance of themselves or others.
- Somatic pain like headaches and stomach aches.

How to help your child when they have fears about their appearance

Show Them How Strong and Capable They Are

Notice all the impressive things your child can do with their body. Are they a good climber? Are they very dextrous and capable with delicate things? Do they have a great memory?

A good eye for colours and fashion? A good ear for catching tunes? Are they brave and not scared of heights? Do they cuddle their siblings softly and with kindness?

Help them add more activities that are good for the body and mind and help them gain even more skills and reasons to be proud of what their amazing body can do.

If you find yourself wanting to comment on your child's appearance, try to focus on what their body can *do* – its health and fitness – rather than how it *looks*.

Find Them Things to Do With Their Body That Make Them Feel Happy, Safe and Connected to Themselves and Others

In addition to feeling strong and capable, you can also work on helping your child feel calm and comfortable in their own skin. Try the following:

- Use safe physical contact like hand-holding, cuddling, massage, secret handshakes and hand-clapping games to increase your child's oxytocin, making them feel loved and liked.
- Show children how to enjoy relaxing and how to listen to their body when it's tired and needs a break.
- Help them find things that make their body feel good and special – for example, painting nails, massage, face paint, moisturising and skin care, yoga, meditation or EFT tapping.
- Make art or be creative.

Loudly Praise the Appearance of Diverse Bodies and Looks

As you watch TV as a family or walk around in public places, comment positively on different kinds of bodies that you see. Praise different styles of hair, shapes and size of bums and tums and the different way that people dress. Also try to notice bodies and shapes of bodies that look like your child's and say calmly how nice they are too.

Some children or teens will find a direct compliment can make them feel uncomfortable or vulnerable, but just knowing you like a body similar to theirs may be enough to help them receive your positive confirmation joyfully.

Try to Find Friends That Look Different to Your Family

Think about your friendship group. If you realise all your friends look just like you, consider the idea that this may be a limiting and constricting factor to your child seeing and appreciating diverse shapes, sizes, skin shades, hair types, builds and bodies. Praise and admire all sorts of lovely vibrant people, including the very old, differently abled and the very young, in front of your family.

Add Body Positive Books to Your Collection

I have seen children's faces light up, their shoulders drop and their breathing regulate when they finally see a character that looks like them receiving compassion and love in a book or magazine. A wide variety of excellent books about body positivity are available. Choose the one that suits your child.

Read books illustrating the beauty in different sizes, skin colours, hair types and ability and see how liberating it can be for your child – and you too!

Change Your Language About Food and Exercise

I have heard many people, usually women, asking for a 'skinny latte' in front of their children and commenting in their earshot about how 'bad' they have been for eating too much, consuming 'fattening' food or not going to the gym.

Your child needs to know they are not bad for eating something yummy, however many calories it contains. There is no such thing as a 'bad' food or a person who is 'bad' for eating a particular food. Food is both fuel and a pleasure. You don't want your child to feel guilty or self-conscious about eating. Even if you are caught up in a vicious cycle of eating and loathing yourself for eating too much of the 'wrong' food, you don't want your child to share your negative experience. Take active steps to protect your child from the misery and guilt you have experienced around food, calories, weight and body image. Making a difference in the way you think and speak about food and eating will not only change the way you feel about yourself, but also your children's idea of their body identity. If you are focusing on the skinny-ness of something, your children will know it is skinny-ness you prize rather than health, strength or wellbeing. Stressing that only very slim people are attractive – even if you have been brought up to believe it – puts a potentially painful focus on an unattainable standard of beauty that is a pressure on you and difficult and worrying for them.

> **Firework idea**
>
> **For most children under fifteen, there will be some cyclical bodily changes. For example, they may have a part of the year where they are rounder and have a bigger tummy and then you may notice that suddenly they seem like they have been rolled out with a rolling pin! These cycles of roundness and leanness can go on until after puberty, so remember to wait calmly for their next growth spurt before worrying about their shape and size.**

Eat as a Family

Eating meals as a family is wonderful for children's well-being:

- It gives families a touchstone to reconnect after the day apart.
- It's a chance to talk and eat calmly where everybody can have their time to share.

- It's an opportunity for children to see eating taking place calmly and enjoyably without pressure.
- It's a chance to try new food.
- It's a place to copy table manners.
- It's an arena for practising social skills and learning to read social cues.
- It's a chance for everyone to put down their devices and be present.
- It's an opportunity to enjoy food and feel the social side of eating.

If eating as a family doesn't fit easily into your daily routine, try to increase the number of times you eat as a team. You don't have to lay a table formally. You don't even need to have space for a table. The point is to be together, chatting, catching up and enjoying nourishing food.

Enjoy Food and Physical Activity Publicly

Studies in 2007, 2016 and 2018 showed that children tended to embrace a healthier lifestyle after seeing parents, particularly fathers, actively engaging in sport and eating healthy meals. The idea is that seeing your role model enjoying food, eating a varied balanced diet and making exercise a fun and important part of their lives helps children find this behaviour appealing and easy to copy.

Find a sport or an activity to get you and your family off the sofa and physically active. Tell your child you are all going to have fun together as a family and get them enthusiastically involved. Showing positivity around being active instils a positive attitude in children over time.

Similarly, eating healthily and enjoying fresh fruit and vegetables, cooking together from scratch sometimes, growing salad leaves then picking and nibbling them, makes children open to doing the same.

Get smiling, munching and moving!

Teach Media Literacy Skills

Our children are bombarded by advertising, TV programmes and social media with a heavy emphasis on one type of body as the most desirable. For girls, we could call her Barbie and for boys we could call him Ken. It is vital and useful to make sure your children know almost 100 per cent of these perfect-looking images have been doctored in some way. Explain to your child about face-tuning and filters. You must make a point of teaching your children the skills to see the reality behind each photo, reel and advert, helping them realise that no one looks the way they do on social media, even at the moment the photograph is taken. Kate Winslet, the Oscar-winning actress and star of *Titanic*, is very clear and honest about this. She says she never looks anything like her heavily edited and computer-enhanced pictures, even on the day they are being taken. Lighting, make-up, hair extensions, filters, retouching all make her look like a very different version of her real self. No one has a flat tummy, a perfect hair day or clear skin all the time and that's OK.

If you give your children the information needed to strip back this view of perfection, their knowledge will protect them against what can feel very much like a constant bombardment of attacks on their self-esteem.

Every so often, choose a photo or video you have seen that is clearly retouched. Show it to your child and ask them what they notice.

- Which part of what they have seen is real?
- Which parts are fake, or manipulated by computers, lighting, make-up, retouching or all those techniques?
- How do you know?
- What kinds of changes might have been made to this content?
- Why do you think they would choose to do that?
- What do you think their choices are meant to tell us about bodies?
- Do you agree?
- What would be better?
- Who makes content that fits better to what you think about bodies?

Speak Fairly About Your Body and Help Them Do the Same

On days when your body is bigger, achy or bloated, talk about your body and how well it serves you, how grateful to it you are even if it doesn't feel at peak performance every minute of every day. Tell your child you are listening to your body with kindness. It might need rest, food, vitamins, a bracing walk, a trip to the doctor or dentist or just a relaxing bubble bath. You will do your best in life to respect and appreciate and care for your body because you need it to go on serving you brilliantly so you can carry on having fun with your beloved family.

For example: when you pull on your jeans and they are too tight, you might have said unthinkingly, 'Oh, I'm so fat! I'm like a whale! I can't even fit into my favourite jeans. It's a diet for me from today.' Choose instead to speak to yourself kindly and set a healthier example to your child. Say, 'Oh, my body is telling me it doesn't want to be constricted by my old jeans. Today I'm going to wear something more comfortable and tomorrow maybe I'll go shopping for some trousers that fit me better.'

If you speak and act kindly on behalf of your body, you model the same empathetic behaviour to your children.

Build Self-esteem in Other Areas

If you have noticed your child's self-esteem is diminishing due to body anxiety, find other activities and ways to show them their worth. What do they enjoy? Focus on that. Stop commenting on their looks and shift focus to activities you know they love and are guaranteed to showcase their talent and capability. Use your energy to build your child up whenever you can to establish a secure sense of self-worth. 'Look at that fabulous cupcake/drawing/kind message/goal! Wow! You amaze me.'

Firework idea

Use social media to reinforce the uplifting message of body positivity and diversity. I recommend teaching songs to younger children about loving yourself and your body. Try 'I Love My Body' by Mother Moon, 'The Positive Affirmation Song' by Super Sema and 'If I Were a Fish' by Corook. The internet can be worrying, but it is well worth remembering it's a useful tool and we can wield it to bring us kindness and positivity to share with our children!

How to help yourself feel less concerned about your child's appearance

Remember your child will get their vision of themselves from YOU. Just because you may be consumed by negative feelings about your body does not mean your child has to experience the same miserable emotions about theirs.

How can you recalibrate your opinions until you can be positive about your body and your child's? All it takes is finding a new angle to change the way you see a situation.

Think about which of these angles might help you release yourself and your child from body-image anxiety.

The 'Don't Pass on Your Pain' Angle

If you have been brought up by a parent who made you feel that you were too fat, too thin, too dark, too short, your hair was too frizzy, or that your appearance was inadequate in any other way, you will have been conditioned over time to believe what they told you was true. Society and other people might well have confirmed their view. So, every time your dress didn't zip up, you were told off for eating too much, you didn't use the hot brush to flatten your hair or you left the house without make-up, you were made to feel awful and flooded with self-loathing.

As a parent, I know you would do anything to protect your child from pain. You wouldn't think twice about donating your kidney to them if they needed it or even taking a bullet for them.

This is your chance to make a genuine effort to help your child. You can be part of the reason they are in pain and tormented by body-image anxiety or you can work your hardest to liberate them from those destructive feelings. You can release them from internal and external criticism by working on your own body positivity, focusing on their kindness and creativity, not what they look like, and helping your child to find their special light and happiness.

The Feminist Angle

Whether you are a man or a woman or identify more fluidly, we can all benefit from a bit of feminism and equality. Every human being should be allowed to look the way they do and be the person they are with pride. Letting yourself be limited or defined by society leads to the opposite of the inclusive, diverse, understanding world we are trying to create.

Whether our sons are being pressured to be muscular or our daughters are pressured to be skinny, we can be a force in the world that makes it a more hospitable, friendlier, less judgemental place for our children and empowers them to fulfil their potential.

We can all advocate for fairer beauty standards, better representation for all body types and an understanding of what is healthy for every size, shape and age.

Be the change you want to see in your child's world and future!

The 'Life Well-lived' Angle

When you look back at your life and when your child looks back at theirs, will you be saying, 'I shouldn't have eaten that cake on that sunny day in Brighton'? Will you be saying, 'That year I was a size 8 was the best of my life'?

NO!!!

You will be wishing you had focused less on the opinions of others, travelled more, experienced all that life had to offer and loved yourself and others truly and without embarrassment.

Make those changes now and allow yourself to know you did all you could to enjoy your time on this planet and you set the best example to enable your child to do the same.

The 'Set Your Life Up Right' Angle

You may not be able to silence the voice in your head telling you that you or your child should look a certain way, but you can find a way to ensure that your family enjoys the kind of life that supports health and happiness, and you can substitute a fairer, more loving voice instead.

You can add health to your life by finding activities you love and fitting them into your schedule, with the ability to adapt and change depending on what you are going through. You can learn to cook healthier food and prioritise nourishment and variety. Show your child how you have set up your life to increase your energy, self-care and overall happiness.

The 'Every Body is Beautiful' Angle

It may sound cheesy, but it's true, everybody and every body is beautiful. The amazing fact that you exist and there will never be another you living in a world like this is a miracle.

You are special! You have a light in you no one else could spark! It's very hard to see it in yourself, particularly when you are exhausted from the responsibility and worry of parenting. However, you possess the power to be proud of or ashamed of your body and now is the time to start loving yourself and showing your child how beautiful they are – every day.

The 'Your Body, Not Theirs – Who Cares!' Angle

Teach yourself and your child to understand, 'It's your body, not theirs – SO WHO CARES!' No one should get to tell you what you should look like or who you should be. So don't let them. If you feel good, you are good. If you like it like that, it's perfect.

If you can be in love with you, that's all you need, and your child will be inspired by how few BLEEPS you give and how your confidence is what people notice about you first. Be a badass mother or father – literally!

The 'Unconditional Love' Angle

This one is not an angle; it's a way to live. You know that what your children want from you, in exactly the same way that you wanted from your parents, is to feel you love and like them, no matter what – unconditionally.

If part of your ability to give your child unconditional love is squashed by your need for them to look different, you are likely to ruin the feeling entirely.

What do you think unconditional love would have improved about your childhood and your relationships now?

As parents, shouldn't we aim to work on ourselves until our children get the best chance at feeling well and truly good enough?

When to seek help for your child with body issues

Seek professional help if you've noticed your child's symptoms increasing and they are now exhibiting any of the following behaviours:

- Eating in a more worrying way including noticeable binge-ing and purging and restrictive eating patterns.
- Losing or gaining weight in a rapid or visible way.
- Any sign of self-harm.
- Increased social isolation.

What support is available for children struggling with body anxiety?

- Your GP.
- Eating disorder and body image specialist psychologists or psychotherapists.
- School support groups.
- Charities such as Beat, Be Body Positive, the Be Real campaign, Health for Teens.

- Counselling and therapy to build self-esteem.
- Hypnotherapy and EFT tapping to fight feelings of anxiety and loss of control.
- Parent support groups.

Books to help your child with body anxiety		
Children	**Teens**	**Adults**
More of Me to Love: A Book About Body Confidence and Body Positivity for Children by Jade Maitre *Lovely* by Jess Hong *We Are Little Feminists: Hair* by Brook Sitgraves Turner and Archaa Shrivastav *Bodies Are Cool* by Tyler Feder *Everybody Has a Body* by Molli Jackson Ehlert *Laxmi's Mooch* by Shelly Anand *The Big Bath House* by Kyo Maclear and Gracey Zhang *Beautifully Me* by Nabela Noor *Brontorina* by James Howe	*A Kids Book About Body Image* by Rebecca Alexander *Every Body: A First Conversation About Bodies* by Megan Madison, Jessica Ralli and Tequitia Andrews *Karma Khullar's Mustache* by Kristi Wientge *Love Your Body* by Jessica Sanders *A Smart Girl's Guide to Liking Herself – Even on the Bad Days* by Laurie Zelinger *Taking Up Space* by Alyson Gerber *Smile* by Raina Telgemeier *Starfish* by Lisa Fipps	*More Than a Body: Your Body Is an Instrument, Not an Ornament* by Lexie Kite and Lindsay Kite *Good Girls Don't Get Fat: How Weight Obsession is Messing Up Our Girls and How We Can Help Them Thrive Despite It* by Robyn J. A. Silverman

Her Body Can by Katie Crenshaw and Ady Meschke *Eyes That Kiss in the Corners* by Joanna Ho *Dancing in the Wings* by Debbie Allen	*The Body Image Book for Girls: Love Yourself and Grow Up Fearless* by Charlotte Markey	

Fourteen

Help! My Child's Anxiety About the Future is Giving Me Anxiety!

What are the very real fears hiding behind this anxiety?

- The fear you will not be able to care for yourself.
- The fear you could die.
- The fear you could be left alone.
- The fear you could be a social outcast.
- The fear you will not be looked after.
- The fear you might become ill and not know how to help yourself.
- The fear the world is not safe.

Anaya had an overprotective mother. Her mum was an anxious and highly capable woman who worried about everything. She put enormous energy and effort into all she did to stave off her fear that she would be exposed as incapable. Mum was part of all Anaya's childhood activities. She was the Brown Owl in her Brownie troop and a governor at her school. She even rewrote Anaya's GCSE and A-level coursework.

Anaya came to see me when she began having panic attacks after receiving an invitation to interview for her dream university in her final year of school. She cried uncontrollably at night-time and was now saying she didn't want to go to university despite being on track to gain a place at Oxford to study history, a subject she had always loved.

When our sessions started, it was almost impossible to get her mum to leave. She wanted to sit in every week. She would say she was listening to a podcast and then occasionally answer a question I had just asked Anaya, following up by saying, 'Don't mind me!'

One day, when Anaya's dad dropped her off and didn't accompany her into our session, I took my chance to work out what was troubling Anaya. My hunch was that she was choosing not to go to university as a way of punishing her mother for interfering in and controlling every aspect of her life.

I couldn't have been more wrong.

Once her mother was not listening, Anaya said, 'Who am I? I have no idea. My mother tells me how to do everything, including what I like, what I don't like, what I should eat, when I should go to bed, even when I should go to the loo. If I leave my mother's side to go to university, I will DIE. I won't know if I'm hungry or ill. I won't know how to do anything. The other students will notice I don't know how to do anything. No one will want to be friends with me. *I* don't want to be friends with me.'

I realised Anaya lacked confidence in her ability to survive outside her family home, away from her mum. She felt that her mother was capable and she herself was incapable. She feared that without her mother controlling and organising every detail of her life, she wouldn't cope and she would fail and be all alone.

That was our starting point. From there we did the following:

1. We worked hard to find out who she was.
2. We talked through how to listen to her body for cues for hunger and other sensations.
3. We worked on the skills needed to care for herself alone.
4. We practised social skills.
5. We worked to find joy and reclaim the things she had once loved.
6. We used the 'homework' I set – something I almost never do – as an excuse to get her mum to take a step back but also to get her to teach her the things she needed to know.
7. I helped her to see what a talented, kind and creative person she was.
8. We started getting excited about what HER life could look like and what adventures she could enjoy.

And then she did it . . . all by herself!

What is so scary about the future for our children?

Whether the goal is leaving home, starting a new job or taking on responsibility, many children begin to feel fearful about the next phase of their lives.

This time of life is anxiety-inducing because:

- Human beings have an innate understanding that separating from our caregivers is dangerous. This is certainly the case when we are babies, but becomes less and less true as we get older. However, as survival is our primary goal, older children still feel that without their parents to protect and guide them, things could go badly wrong.
- Being given more responsibility is scary. What if you forget to brush your teeth, wake up for work or budget your money properly? The consequences can be dire. Knowing the buck stops with you for the first time is intimidating.
- The skills children need to acquire as they become adults take time to learn and master. When their first wash dyes everything pink or they fail their driving test, it dents their confidence and makes them anxious that they'll never get the hang of adult life.
- Fear of failure or letting people down can freeze them in an anxious state, stopping them having another try at a task that defeated them initially.
- Lack of control or a feeling of overwhelming uncertainty can derail young people. They are brimming with questions about the world, the office, romance, sex and education, but they don't yet have any answers.

A young person quickly realises their school, parents, family and friends have been a buffer, making life easier for them. They were told reassuring things they hoped would be true. Anything is possible! Work hard and you'll get there! Be yourself and they will love you! Unfortunately, in practice, these comforting sentiments don't seem quite as cut and dried.

How do you know if your child is scared of the future?

- They seem to be more panicked than previously about exams, starting a new phase or changes in their relationships. They talk about those things frequently with trepidation.
- They may be more irritable than usual.
- They may be avoiding talking about the end of school, the summer, applications, their job start date, etc.
- They may be delaying making decisions like signing up for halls of residence, applying for jobs or packing up to leave.
- They may be experiencing sleep changes like insomnia, massively oversleeping to put off decision-making, or having nightmares.
- They have low self-esteem and regularly say how poor they are at doing things. When you explain you think they are good or talented, they disagree.
- They may suffer somatic complaints like persistent stomach aches, tummy problems or headaches.
- They suddenly want to be near you all the time.
- Alternatively, they might want to separate from you and hardly speak to you in preparation for leaving.
- They ask for reassurance all the time.

- You notice increased checking or organising in a way that seems all-consuming.
- They withdraw from social activities.

How do we help our children feel better prepared for what is to come?

Build Their Confidence by Teaching Them Life Skills

Start by thinking about your own life. Which skills have been most useful – in your teenage years, your first year living outside the family home, your first job or your daily life? What can you teach your child before they move on that will best equip them to manage what comes next?

Here are some ideas:

- Cleaning – how to change your sheets, do the laundry, clean a kitchen and a bathroom, how to stay on top of mess.
- Home maintenance – how to change a light bulb, put in a nail, build a flatpack, change a plug.
- First aid – for cuts, burns, choking, how to make an emergency call.
- Cooking – simple recipes, basic nutrition, food hygiene, how to build the microbiome.
- Good manners – being respectful to everyone, always aiming to help others.

- Financial skills – budgeting, saving and investing, understanding credit.
- Knowing your own worth – consent, self-esteem and knowing your own values.
- Hard work – growth mindset, stamina, asking for help.
- Critical thinking – being media critical, resourcefulness and practical decision-making skills.

You may have come up with many more.

Now think about how you can pass these skills on to your child before they move on to the next part of their lives.

You can write a list and tick off each skill. Let your child know this is something you are accomplishing together so they can start the next phase of their lives prepared.

Tell them you are wondering how you can help them acquire the right skills. Ask what 'adulting' they'd like to be better at before they go?

Help Them Prepare for What's in Store

Give your child as much information as possible or help them find the best option for them. Anxiety is reduced if we are given the right information to answer our nagging internal questions: what will it be like? Where is it? Who will be there? What will I need? How is it different from something I've done before? If they are leaving home to go to university, try the following:

- Look through the university website together.
- Find someone who goes to that university/works at that place to talk to.
- Use online forums to ask questions.
- Talk through what you both know about work or university.
- Look up travel links to get home or to university.
- Talk through what you think they might pack and why.
- Ask if they have everything they think they will need.
- Go through student finance with them.
- Look through job listings in their university city with them if you know finances will be tight.
- Ask, 'What do you think will be different from what you have done before?' Address fears and misinformation, and supply what your child needs.

Your Child Can Change Their Mind

It's a common misconception that children should know what they want to do with their lives by the time they are 16 and choose their GCSEs. It's nonsense and unhelpful. People happily change their minds all the time about their choice of GCSE/A-level subjects, whether they should stay at their school or go to college, what they will study at university, which university they would go to, or whether they should do a post-grad, a gap year or go straight to work. They are all fine! Most are happy!

Make sure your child knows that they can change their mind at any point and you will help them find the right path when or if they need it. Transferring is allowed; changing flats is allowed; starting over is allowed; not liking what you thought you would like is allowed.

Liberate your child by explaining the aim is to make the best decision we can with what we know. Then:

- We try the plan.
- We give it our best shot.
- We give it a little longer to see if we do or don't like it.
- Then we look around for other sensible options if the choice turns out to be wrong for us.

Remind Them They Can Always Come Home

It liberates and relaxes our children if they know that they can always come home and we will always be happy to see them. Home is meant to be a safe place for our children when they are little. Why should that change as they get older? Our adult children should always be able to walk through the door to our homes and shut out the rest of the world. Tell your child your home will always be theirs and you will always be there, happy to help them back on their feet with a bit of TLC.

New Things Are Only New for a Short Time

Remind your child that whenever you start something new or go somewhere unfamiliar, it seems odd, different, difficult and scary. Soon you learn where the loo is, how to get from place A to place B and find someone to have lunch with and the place becomes familiar and unthreatening. Newcomers quickly turn into regulars.

In my experience, it takes about three to four weeks until you are semi-established somewhere new and it starts to feel normal to be there.

Remind Them You Will Always Be There if They Need You

As your child prepares to leave home, plan a conversation with them where you say something along these lines:

> My darling, I know you are all grown up and you are capable, loveable and ready for your next adventure . . . but I just want to say, as I'm sure you know, I am always here if you need me. I cannot do magic, but I can be here at the end of the phone and I will help you with anything. I know how to solve most problems. I will always be there in an emergency. I am your parent and I hope I'm also a friend and sometimes an expert! So, ask me. Call me and I'll always be pleased to hear from you and make time to do everything I can to help, even if it is just to listen.

I don't think there's a young person in the world who wouldn't feel comforted and relieved by this clear moment of connection, care and promise.

Help Your Child Be the Architect of Their Own Life

We can all see how quickly life passes. We all have dreams. There are places we wish we had visited, ambitions we wish we had fulfilled and ideas we wish we had acted upon. What we would really like for our children is long, adventurous, beautiful, full lives.

If we make our children feel as if we don't trust them to explore or they aren't good enough to set off on their own, we are limiting their achievements and making them fearful.

Sit down with your child and ask, 'What are your dreams? Where would you travel if you could go anywhere? What does a life well lived look like to you? What do you need to know, have, be to live the life you can imagine?' They might need financial help. However, it is probably your opinion, advice, empathy, enthusiasm, googling and listening capacity that will open or shut life's doors for your children.

Whatever their dreams or their personalities, show them they can be in charge, make their own plans and take their own risks and you believe they can go anywhere they want to go.

Set Them Up With a Healthy Timetable They Can Fall Back On

I call it the 'self-care checklist', but it is a way to help our children to be sure they are doing everything their bodies need to provide the energy and brain chemicals to thrive. It reminds our children to prioritise looking after themselves. It's great as an everyday structure for life and also works well as a short intervention to help when our children are having a low mental health moment away from home.

> **Firework idea**
>
> **This is a very easy way to boost your child's mental health from afar. Take a photo of things you think would help your child stay focused, boost their mood or engage them socially, then email it over or print it out and surprise them with a positive bit of snail mail!**

Aim for at least three ticks a week in at least five boxes.

Saskia Joss

Date _____

	Monday	Tuesday	Wednesday	Thursday	Friday	Weekend
Slept for more than six hours						
Had a bath/shower						
Got dressed						
Ate healthily						
Saw a friend						
Went outside in nature for more than thirty mins						
Did some exercise						
Did something to make myself feel better						
Ticked something off my to-do list						

Why does letting our children become adults give us anxiety?

- It reminds us we are also getting older.
- It makes us feel we haven't done enough to prepare our child to be safe without us.
- It may bring up questions about who we are when we no longer have to focus on parenting all the time.
- It may bring up questions about our romantic relationship now we haven't got our child to concentrate on.
- You might feel you have no control over your child, which might make you feel out of control yourself.

So what can we do about it?

The key is to maintain respect, kindness and connection with our children no matter what they do, who they become or where they live.

When we bring our babies home from the hospital or on those long sleepless nights or hard days of potty training, we cannot imagine there will ever be a day when our children exist without us. As they go through their teen years, pull away and spend more time with their friends, we begin to see they will not consult us over every decision, but we are still profoundly shocked when they are so self-sufficient we don't even know what they have eaten, what time they went to bed and who they are spending time with.

Some parents will try to stop the process by holding on more tightly, calling more often and expressing stronger opinions to try to stay relevant and in control. This can lead to adult children holding back information from their parents or pulling away even further.

I recommend that if you want to maintain a lasting relationship, the key is to be excited for your adult child. Be pleased for their wins and console them for their losses. Know there will be phases where they need us more and some where they need us less, but always try to meet them with kindness and respect.

We want our children to love and be loved, to try new things, to travel, take risks, believe in themselves and have the courage to try their utmost to make at least some of their dreams come true.

If they are happy, be relieved and celebrate. If they are not, offer your ear, time, support and advice if asked for. You can be proud you gave all the kindness and love you could.

What support is available for children who are anxious about the future?

Therapeutic support for adolescents or young adults can be empowering if they are facing a big life change such as leaving home or starting a new job. Explore the following options:

- Therapy with an adolescent specialist
- Art therapy
- Person-centred therapy
- EMDR (see page 203)
- CBT (see page 41)

- Hypnotherapy
- Online forums about starting work or going to university
- Speak to your university about a peer mentor or what plans they have for orientation or tours around campus
- Help your child find pre-work online courses. Try Future-Learn, Udemy, Coursera, LinkedIn Learning, Barclays LifeSkills or Founders4Schools
- Mental health apps can keep young people focused and supported without the need for more expensive support
- If your child is very worried about starting work, look into a few sessions with a career coach or online seminars about entering their field of work from places like The Coaching Academy, National Careers Service or PushFar

Books to help your child with anxiety about the future
The Defining Decade: Why Your Twenties Matter and How to Make the Most of Them Now by Meg Jay
Brave Not Perfect: Fear Less, Fail More and Live Bolder by Reshma Saujani
You Don't Understand Me: The Young Woman's Guide to Life by Dr Tara Porter
Life Skills for Young Adults: How to Manage Money, Find a Job, Stay Fit, Eat Healthy and Live Independently by Ferne Bowe
How to Adult, a Practical Guide: Advice on Living, Loving, Working, and Spending Like a Grown-Up by Jamie Goldstein
How to Thrive with Adult ADHD: 7 Pillars for Focus, Productivity and Balance by Dr James Kustow
They Don't Teach This at School: Essential Knowledge to Tackle Everyday Challenges by Myleene Klass
The Young Autistic Adult's Independence Handbook by Haley Moss

Fifteen

Help! My Child's Gender Anxiety is Giving Me Anxiety!

What are the very real fears hiding behind this anxiety?

- The fear you are wrong or doing something wrong by being yourself.
- The fear you are different from others in a negative way.
- The fear you will be cast out by family or friends.
- The fear you will never be accepted as yourself.
- The fear you have disappointed your family.

This chapter was written with the support of Orla Muriel Blakelock, a trauma-informed integrative therapist living in Brighton. They work primarily with the queer community and regularly support adults to navigate their gender identity and transition. They have worked in mental health since 2009 and for organisations such as Gendered Intelligence, Stonewall, Bipolar UK, the Advocacy Project and the NHS.

When do young people start considering their gender?

Young people think about their gender when their inclinations, thoughts and feelings do not match the expectation

349

of the gender that they have been assigned at birth. This could happen in relation to who they play with, which toys they like or what they want to wear, but deeper consideration and emotions about gender usually occur at the start of puberty.

A 2008 study showed that most gender-non-conforming children had begun to discuss their awareness of differences by the time they were three years old.

However, children assigned female at birth (AFAB) often find developing breasts or starting their periods definite markers of womanhood. Those with a feeling of difference will often find puberty a watershed moment, leading to considerable anxiety and distress.

Puberty brings those assigned male at birth (AMAB) pressure to behave in a 'typical' masculine way which, in those with feelings of difference, can lead to anxiety, distress and a feeling of social segregation.

And for those who are intersex (those with both kinds of body parts), puberty can lead to severe confusion and anxiety.

What can parents do to support children as they start to explore their gender?

The key is to keep communication open and to follow your child's lead.

When shopping for clothes or toys, make sure that if your

child chooses something they love, you aim to show your approval with your face and body language and continue to be positive about it when they are in earshot.

Be the kind of parent who makes a safe space for all self-expression. Comment kindly and without judgement about people's gender differences on TV or when you meet them. Your calm and kind response to others will show your child how you would receive them if they came to you to discuss their gender-based worries.

How can parents help constructively when children begin to explore gender in a more visible way?

The key is to work on your own feelings about gender, about clothes and haircuts and about expectations. Think about what your parents, teachers and religious leaders told you about gender. You were probably told what was 'normal' or 'abnormal', 'right' or 'wrong', 'bad' and 'evil' or 'good' and 'righteous'. Now think about the child you love. They are not abnormal, wrong, bad or evil. They are simply themselves, trying to carve out an identity they can flourish in and feel comfortable with. If you appreciate your child is doing their best to navigate their way through a tough and testing situation without examples or role models, it will have less impact when your son wants nail varnish or your daughter asks for a shorter haircut.

As a parent, we know all we want is for our child to find life easy and to be happy. If they want to wear something or play with something that will make them happy, we have to work to dislodge the preconceptions that make their choices problematic. Our work on ourselves will make our homes an easier and more encouraging place for our kids to be themselves no matter what they are going through.

> **Firework idea**
>
> **A study from 2009 showed that children who felt extremely accepted when sharing their gender identity with their families showed a 92 per cent likelihood of feeling happy in adulthood. It was also seen to directly protect against depression and suicidality.**

What are the signs and symptoms a child may be having gender anxiety?

These look similar to the symptoms of other anxieties. Your child might withdraw or be emotionally volatile. They may become depressed and not want to engage socially. They might have somatic pain like headaches and stomach aches. They might become overwhelmed at times that bring this anxiety to the fore, like getting dressed or having to socialise in a certain way. You may not even be sure exactly what is worrying them.

Orla's suggestion is: 'When, as a parent, you are trying to establish what could be behind your child's anxiety and thinking, "Could it be school, social anxiety or family worries?", add gender anxiety to the list.'

It doesn't have to be top of the list, but bear it in mind. Ask questions to give your child the chance to talk through their identity and whether what they wear or how they look fits their sense of who they are and who they want to be.

Let's talk about gender dysphoria and how you can tell if your child has it

Gender dysphoria is the feeling of confusion and distress when a person's gender identity doesn't match the gender that they were assigned at birth and brought up with. It may start with emotional symptoms – for example, seeming emotionally overwhelmed, angry or low. Children may suddenly struggle to get dressed in a way that they haven't previously. Imagine living with the sensation that how you feel and how you look do not match. Gender dysphoria is highly distressing and can make a child feel that everything in their life is wrong.

Gender dysphoria is all-consuming and can take children to a confusing and low place. It can make children or adults feel very isolated. Try to listen to your child's experience without criticism. They may look or seem the same, but that is not how they feel. Help keep children connected to you and others who understand them by keeping them in as regular a schedule as possible and consider visiting a gender-affirming doctor with experience of dysphoria, or speaking to a charity. Focus on finding

---

like-minded people who can understand this very difficult period in your child's life.

Pay attention to your feelings when you get pronouns
wrong. Could YOU be experiencing shame or embarrassment?

Shame and queerness sadly go hand in hand for many of
us. We have been trained to feel that queerness and transi-
tioning are wrong. If you have never felt gender dysphoria
or even questioned your own gender, it can be extremely
hard to fully empathise. When you understand your pro-
gramming or misunderstanding is based on outdated
gender norms, prejudice or bigotry, you can do your best
to release yourself to support the child you love dearly.

Firework idea

**If your child has asked to use different pronouns, help
them see you are on their team and supportive of who
they are by politely and quickly correcting those who
use the wrong ones to describe them. It can be very
tiring to have to keep explaining yourself and it's a
clear gesture of care and acceptance.**

Once your child has told you they identify as non-binary or trans, what are the first steps a parent should take to help anxiety?

Primarily, we talk about social transition, which is the first stage of presenting yourself in a way that matches your internal identity.

That usually means discussion of pronouns, the name they want to be called and a focus on aesthetics. We want to make sure our child has all the support they need at home, within the extended family and at school so they can be the person they feel they truly are.

It shouldn't be expensive to give them what they need to try to bring out this part of their identity. This is their first attempt at finding who they want to be in the world on their own terms. Their interpretation of their needs may change later, but it is important to listen and help them turn the idea they have of themselves inside their heads into the individual they project in real life.

Your child may also need time and support to test out a new name that fits who they are now. Some young people will feel that as their name no longer matches their idea of themselves, it's a name they no longer wish to hear again. The term 'dead name' – a phrase used to describe the name they used to go by – seems drastic and can be upsetting for the parents who chose and used that name all this time, as it implies that the person you knew is dead. However, for most people exploring gender, they are battling against the trauma and confusion of gender dysphoria and having a new name can often be the first step to starting their new, more comfortable life.

To use your new name socially or at school, there should be no need for any formal process or paperwork. If children are allowed to ask a teacher to call them by a nickname, they should be able to change the name they go by at school without any issue.

If your child would like to have their new name on their passport or medical documents, they will likely need a deed poll, which is a legally binding document for anyone in the UK who wants to formally change their name. This can be after marriage or family change or because someone would like a new name and is not exclusive to trans and non-binary people. As of writing this book, the service costs just under £50. You can then send the deed poll document to the passport office or doctor's surgery to start the process of having your child's new name used officially.

Talk to your child's school and other key people in their world. You can ask your child how they want their new information to be shared and who they want to be made aware of their situation. Do they want to be part of the conversation or would they like you to tell people on their behalf?

The aim is to be an advocating ally for your child and work to make sure they have what they need to feel safe and supported everywhere they go.

If you have difficult personal feelings about your child exploring or changing their gender, what should you do?

Everyone has digested some level of information about gender. I've met families using they/them pronouns for their children from birth who still struggle at points to support changes in their child's gender and presentation. We all have feelings about roles or looks attributed to men and women. We have all been brought up in a mainly heteronormative, binary society and we will all carry some of that with us despite the work we have done on ourselves.

Obviously, cisgendered/heterosexual people will have done far less delving into their gender or sexuality than someone who is gender non-conforming or trans ('cisgendered' means someone whose gender identity matches their sex assigned at birth). Having a gender-questioning child may lead a parent to question themselves and what they know.

There is no shame in struggling with your own feelings at the same time as doing your best to help your child. Find a therapist, join a support group, speak to a more progressive religious community leader, find a supportive friend and see if you can work on ways to love and support your child while valuing your principles.

One question that often arises is whether you should conceal your issues in order to protect your child, while you work on your grief or negative feelings. The answer is that your child will receive the message subconsciously. They will notice an incongruence in the way you respond to them. The idea is to be honest in the kindest way you can.

That might sound like: 'I love you no matter what. I've always loved you and will always love you. Your gender exploration has brought up lots of questions for me too and you have inspired me to work on myself and what I know about gender. It might take me a bit of time to understand all the new information about you and about me, but that's my plan and that's what I'm going to do.'

Which other issues can increase anxiety for trans and non-binary children?

Social Issues

There tend to be more social issues for trans people. They can be subjected to bullying or even abuse. You will need to keep a close eye on your child's school to make sure support systems and anti-bullying protocols are in place. Knowledge and understanding are improving and many schools now support trans and non-binary youths with kindness and professionalism.

The Additional Impact of Faith and Community

Trans and non-binary young people may feel excluded from their place of worship and other community activities. Consider how being talked about or not feeling allowed or accepted somewhere they used to go regularly might feel. If necessary, act as a shield to protect your child from religious or judgemental community members. Your child will flourish when they are included in a community that understands them. Finding that community can be even more difficult for people of colour and for those with disabilities and neurodivergence.

Let your child know they are an integral part of your family no matter what and you are determined to do the best you can to help them find their tribe outside the family too.

Dating

Dating can be complicated for trans and non-binary teenagers. Having to come out as trans to a new partner or having to show your body to another when you have struggled with gender dysphoria can be very difficult. Having good friends and relationships can help children find the right place to talk about these issues, particularly if they don't feel comfortable discussing them with you.

This may also be a time to help your child find a queer-positive therapist who can support them as they begin dating.

Providing Safe Locations at School

More and more schools in the UK offer gender-neutral lavatory facilities. However, if your child's school does not have unisex loos or if your child has been experiencing bullying at school, you may need to contact the school to make sure they can support your child and they feel safe and supported.

When is it time to visit a doctor?

Even at the very beginning of your child's gender exploration, it's useful for parents and children to have support. Speak to your GP about information and other services available to your family and your child. You may be able to find a therapist, support group or charity that can help your child navigate this tricky time.

Much publicity has been given to the number of under-eighteens receiving puberty-blocking medication. In 2023, there were fewer than 100 children in the UK on puberty-blockers. Seek information and professional advice.

What support is available for gender-questioning, trans and non-binary youth?

- Charities and organisations like The Clare Project Gender Construction Kit, Gender Identity Research & Education Society (GIRES), Gendered Intelligence and Mermaids as well as other smaller local charities can provide information and support.

- Support and social groups for trans and non-binary youth can be found all over the UK. Try the group search on the Proud Trust website to find groups near you.
- Online groups and forums can be helpful – though make sure you check the information about being trans your child gets if it might be from an unreliable source.
- Therapeutic support such as art therapy, talking therapy, person-centred therapy or counselling can be really helpful for the exploration and acceptance part of gender identity – make sure to find a trans- and non-binary-affirming and experienced therapist.
- School support such as a gay–straight alliance (a club set up in school for LGBTQIA+ youth and their ally friends) and in-school therapy.

Books to help your child with gender anxiety		
Children	**Teens**	**Adults**
Being You: A First Conversation about Gender by Megan Madison, Jessica Ralli and Anne/Andy Passchier Gender Identity for Kids by Andy Passchier It Feels Good to Be Yourself by Theresa Thorn Julian Is a Mermaid by Jessica Love	The Gender Wheel by Maya Gonzales Sex is a Funny Word: A Book About Bodies, Feelings, and You by Corey Silverberg and Fiona Smyth Melissa by Alex Gino Gracefully Grayson by Ami Polonsky Snapdragon by Kat Leyh	Parenting Beyond Pink and Blue: How to Raise Your Kids Free of Gender Stereotypes by Christina Spears Brown Free to Be: Understanding Kids & Gender Identity by Jack Turban Challenging Gender Stereotypes in the Early Years: Changing the Narrative by Susie Heywood and Barbara Adzajlic

My Shadow Is Purple by Scott Stuart *A House for Everyone: A Story to Help Children Learn About Gender Identity and Gender Expression* by Jo Hirst	*Ana on the Edge* by A. J. Sass *The Other Boy* by M. G. Hennessey *Gender Identity Workbook for Teens: Practical Exercises to Navigate Your Exploration, Support Your Journey, and Celebrate Who You Are* by Andrew Maxwell Triska	*Gender Explained: A New Understanding of Identity in a Gender Creative World* by Dr Diane Ehrensaft and Dr Michelle Jurkiewicz *Raising Them: Our Adventure in Gender Creative Parenting* by Kyl Myers *Childhood Unlimited: Parenting Beyond the Gender Bias* by Virginia Mendez *Talking to Kids about Gender Identity: A Roadmap for Christian Compassion, Civility, and Conviction* by Mark Yarhouse

Sixteen

Help! My Child's Anxiety About Their Sexuality is Giving Me Anxiety!

What are the very real fears hiding behind this anxiety?

- The fear you are wrong or doing something wrong just by being yourself.
- The fear you are different from others in a negative way.
- The fear you will be cast out by family or friends.
- The fear you are going to hell or other religious punishments.
- The fear you have disappointed your family.

This chapter was written with the support of Jamie Crabb, a therapist, lecturer and author who lives in Brighton. He has worked with young people in educational and therapeutic settings for over twenty years. He believes in helping everyone find their authentic self and has practised at charities like Mind, supporting mental health; Diversity & Ability, championing (neuro)Diversity and (dis)Ability inclusion; and the REES Foundation, supporting those who have lived within the care system.

Let's start with a case study from my child therapy practice. One day, I had a call from the mother of a nine-year-old boy.

She asked if I would be able to help her son, Blake, who had been showing signs of anxiety. He regularly had headaches and stomach aches and often looked worried at home and at school. He had a kind and caring family, he had great friends and he was naturally talented at everything sporty and academic. His mum had no idea what had happened and he told her neither did he.

A few weeks into our sessions, Pride month began. I have small decorations that I put up in my therapy room to show all my clients that this is a place where all of them will be accepted. Children as young as seven have started to comment on my rainbow hearts and what they represent, often prompted by lessons they have had at school about Pride and inspirational LGBTQIA+ figures. Blake, however, had not been told about Pride and its history. He went to a Catholic school and came from a religious family. But he did ask me why I had put up rainbow bunting in my room.

I explained that it was because I was an LGBTQIA+ ally and I believe people should proudly be who they are and love who they love and that Pride is an annual celebration of that idea. To my surprise, Blake began to laugh . . . He got the giggles; he couldn't stop laughing. I was shocked. I kindly asked what had tickled him and helped him calm down enough to talk. 'I didn't know you could talk about gay people not in a sad way. Like I thought you could only be disappointed or think it's a sin.' I explained that obviously different people feel different things, but in the UK, it has been legal to get married if you are LGBTQIA+ for a very long time. 'You can marry and celebrate being in love with anyone you want,' I said. 'I think we all want to feel loved and be happy and whether you do that with someone who is the same gender as you or not, feeling safe, happy and loved is all that matters.'

In our next sessions, we spoke more about how that related to his own life, feelings and relationships. He had thought he might be gay as he had wanted to kiss his male friend when they shared a tent on school camp. He hadn't told anyone and had felt very worried he was doing something wrong.

We worked together for most of the year and, after finding a friend at his church who also thought she was a lesbian, he decided he would tell his mum.

He asked if he could tell her in the room with me and we worked out a structure for the conversation. Although his mum had never really spoken to him about queer relationships before, he was about 50 per cent sure that she would be OK with his sexual orientation even though she was religious.

The day came and Blake told his mum that he thought he was gay. His mum was surprised but relieved as she had been very worried about him. The idea that he had worked this out about himself rather than there being something sinister or sad happening to him was, as she said, 'the best reveal I could have asked for'.

Mum helped Blake to work out when it was right to share his information with different family members and friends. She made sure Blake was watched at school by staff so that he wasn't bullied and that any negative attitudes were contained in school. As no other children in his class were talking about their sexual orientation yet, she found him a local support group and helped him find ways to express himself that matched his identity. He told me that knowing he was allowed to be himself and that he didn't have to hide it was all he needed to relax and enjoy himself.

When do children start to notice their sexual orientation?

Early Childhood

In early childhood, children begin to notice their sexual feelings. Boys are aware of their penises becoming erect. Girls notice their genitals are different from their father's and brothers'. Some young children may begin to be aware of differences between themselves and their friends. They might realise, for example, that their responses don't seem to be the same as their friends' when watching a couple kiss in a film. If you are a little girl and your romantic interest is Cinderella, not Prince Charming, it's understandable to feel as if you are out of step with other people's expectations. Children might also begin to develop crushes or early romantic feelings for children of the same gender, which may confuse and worry them.

Adolescence

In adolescence, as hormones rage and sexual desires develop and can become all-consuming, children will realise they are experiencing romantic feelings and sexual desire for one, both or all genders. At this point, children who have been brought up to think of sex as shameful, forbidden or dirty, and those who worry that being attracted to someone of the same sex is wrong, do not feel safe to express their budding sexuality. These young people are gripped by anxiety because they are keeping a secret and fear the truth could be exposed at any time. They fear the nature of their sexual orientation will be considered abnormal, disgusting or shameful.

Their apprehension can be exacerbated by the culture in their particular school. If fellow pupils use the word 'gay' in a pejorative, derogatory way, a child with gay, lesbian or bisexual inclinations understandably thinks that if they were to come out, they would be judged, condemned and ostracised. Naturally, coming to terms with your sexuality is also much more difficult if you believe your parents will be disappointed or disgusted by the discovery.

A study of LGBTQIA+ youth in 1993 revealed that most queer young people have had their first same-gender crush by the time they were ten years old. By the time a similar study was repeated in 2006 and 2009, children reported having their first crush by age seven and these studies showed that on average in 2009, most LGBTQIA+ children had come out to their families by age thirteen.

What are the signs and symptoms that someone is experiencing anxiety about their sexuality?

- Withdrawal from regular social activities.
- Somatic pain such as headaches or stomach aches.
- Negative self-image and low self-esteem.
- Emotional dysregulation.
- Seeming very stressed all the time.
- Being highly critical.
- Obsessing over friendships or feeling lost socially.

How can you show your children that you support and accept them?

Representation and receptiveness to all lifestyles is key and can be done so simply.

- When you are watching TV and see a gay couple, say something positive and human. 'Wow, what a beautiful couple!' Or 'I love it when we see different kinds of couples on TV!'
- When talking about the relationships your child might have getting older, just add in alternative genders: 'When you grow up and find a boyfriend or girlfriend or partner . . .'

- Aim to show that talking about sex and sexuality is not frowned upon but can be done appropriately. This can be done by talking about consent, different kinds of relationships and bodies from when your children begin to notice their own body, at around two years old. You can do that by using appropriate medical terms for body parts, like penis, vagina or vulva. You explain that private parts are private and that means others will not touch them or look at them unless it is your parent or a doctor and, in all cases, they will ask before they do.
- Talk openly about safe touch and how no one is allowed to touch you if it hurts or feels uncomfortable.

Firework idea

Studies in 2016 and 2018 showed that children who had been taught about consent, personal boundaries and the anatomical names for body parts were more likely to engage in safe relationships with adults and children and were more likely to notice, stop and correctly explain dangerous situations with adults.

- You can also add books into your child's collection that show different kinds of representation and relationships. There are so many great books for young kids that show different kinds of families or children both in terms of their likes and dislikes and also their gender and sexual identity.

- If you can make being queer something you talk about as regularly and calmly as you would being straight, you would increase your child's feeling that, if they were to come out, you would accept them as much as you did when you did not know what sexuality they were.

How can you support your child to come to terms with their sexual orientation?

Trying to help your child feel safe and confident enough to talk to you about their sexuality can be difficult because young people are always reluctant to discuss their sexual fantasies or activities with their parents. Make it crystal clear to your child you are not trying to persuade them to reveal details of their sex life. What you do want is to reassure them that they can discuss relationships, dating and the fact that they are attracted to people of their own sex or both sexes with you freely and without fear of judgement.

Let your child know you understand being a young person can be tough. All sorts of unexpected things crop up all the time. You might be offered drugs, drink too much alcohol, have a sexual encounter you regret or fail your driving test. You can't prepare your child for everything that will happen to them, but you will always be there to talk through new experiences, problems or emotions – and sexual orientation is just another part of life. Tell your child, 'I am happy and comfortable talking about friendships, sexuality, gender, romance . . . I've seen it all before. I am not embarrassed by anything you might want to tell or ask me. I am absolutely unshockable. Every teenager needs an adult to help them understand what's going on in their head and heart. I am that person. Whatever comes up that you need or want to chat through, I am in your corner. Or if you find it difficult to speak to me right now, we can find a therapist or mentor if you prefer.'

Let's talk about embarrassment

If you are embarrassed about talking about sex or sexuality, practise discussing it in the mirror by yourself. Practise saying things like:

- 'Whoever you love, the key is that they are kind to you and respect you. I want them to treat you well. Whether they are boys, girls or they are non-binary, I will be happy for you if you are happy.'
- 'When it comes to relationships, any boy or girl would be lucky to have you.'

Think about your child's smiling face as you show them you love them no matter what and how safe and supported they will feel being 100 per cent authentic.

Firework idea

Hold in mind the statistics from a 2009 study that showed the feeling of family support and acceptance directly correlated to positive mental health for LGBTQIA+ adults. Those who felt they had a high level of family support had a 92 per cent likelihood of positive mental health in adulthood and were less likely to be depressed, anxious or suicidal.

When your child comes out

1. Try to be relaxed and do not interrupt them, even if you already suspected.
2. Try to show you are proud of them for telling you something so important.
3. Let them know you love them and this doesn't change that for you.
4. Try not to make it about you; this is their 'coming out' moment.
5. Let them know you are here to listen to anything they feel you should understand about this.
6. Let them know you are happy to help them with any of their next steps, telling other family members (when they are ready), helping them access services for LGBTQIA+ young people or anything else they think they might need.

7. Tell them you will always be here to talk about anything that comes up in their life.
8. Tell them again that you love them and are proud of them.

One child I worked with asked his lovely mum if being gay would stop her loving him. She replied: 'I love you, and nothing you could do or be could stop me.' The child joked, 'What if I killed you?' and the mum replied, 'Well, then I would have to come back and haunt you to show you how much I will always love you!'

After your child has had this conversation with you, check in on them again in the next few days. Coming out can feel like a very big moment and they might need a few days to calm down afterwards.

How can you find support if having a gay child gives you anxiety or makes you feel sad or uncomfortable?

We have all grown up in a heteronormative society. Many of us grew up before gay marriage was legal. Some of us were raised in traditional or religious families. It's hardly surprising that some parents are apprehensive and disappointed at the discovery that their child is gay.

Some parents believe their beloved child is committing a sin and could be punished by God. Some have always dreamed of a traditional wedding for their child and realise that dream may never now come true in the way they imagined.

Finding out your child is LGBTQIA+ may also bring up feelings around your own sexuality. Perhaps you were forbidden from expressing your sexual orientation when we were younger?

If finding out your child is gay gives you anxiety, it's not your fault. We all struggle with differences in life and we have all been brought up in different ways and with value systems or beliefs that are conflicted.

Try your best not to condemn your child or make them responsible for your conflicting emotions. Instead, say something like, 'I'm very proud of you for being able to tell me this. It turns out that finding out about your sexuality has raised interesting thoughts for me. So now I need to do some thinking and learning to make sure I can support you as well as I can.'

Consider joining a parent support group, talking to other friends who have queer children or speaking to a counsellor or therapist for a few sessions to see if they can help you come to terms with the news. How can you be helped to find a way to maintain a loving relationship with your child without feeling you have abandoned your principles?

For further support for parents, try the Families and Friends of Lesbians and Gays (FFLAG).

What do parents need to understand about dating to support their child effectively?

- Only one person in ten is gay so your child may say or feel that the dating pool is small and limited.
- Your child may feel a pressure to adapt the way they dress to fit in with certain groups. Let them know you are fine with their choices. Your child may go through many different looks until they settle on one. Help them have access to hairstyles and clothes that better fit their identity now they are out.
- Your child may need to understand how to have safe sex with men and women. In-school gay sex education is limited. You might need to find out more about queer sex in order to help your child navigate their sex life.
- To meet potential partners, your child may go to queer pubs and clubs which are not only for younger people. Alcohol and drugs may be part of the scene. You may have to talk to your LGBTQIA+ child about alcohol and drugs in more detail and at an earlier age than you expected, just to make sure you have set legal and safe boundaries around them.

Check your child is not being bullied

LGBTQIA+ young people have a higher chance of being bullied or targeted in school, which can make them feel highly anxious and unsafe. It's important to watch out for changes in behaviour, depressive episodes and school refusal. Loneliness is one of the biggest problems facing queer youth. Help your child feel accepted. Help them find their 'queer tribe' (like-minded friends) and other groups that will welcome them.

Consult the section on bullying (see page 158) for further information.

Firework idea

If your child has experienced any behaviour from fellow students that makes them feel scared or uncomfortable, ask your child's school to set up a Gay–Straight Alliance or club for LGBTQIA+ students – or at least provide a safe location where your child and their friends may spend break and lunchtime to take them out of the main playground.

What support is available for young people struggling with anxiety and mental health issues while exploring their sexuality?

- Charities such as Stonewall, Barnardos, Mind, The Proud Trust, Asexual Visibility and Education Network (AVEN), London Friend and the LGBT Foundation provide lots of resources and support for those in the LGBTQIA+ community.

- Speak to your child's school and see what other support they can put in place.
- Go to your GP for support if your child's mental health deteriorates.
- Therapeutic support including art therapy, person-centred therapy or counselling can all be helpful – make sure that the practitioner you choose is LGBTQIA+ affirming and will provide a safe place for them to talk.
- Online forums.
- Online and in-person support groups.
- LGBTQIA+ alliance groups.
- Local youth clubs – use the Proud Trust website's search to find groups close to where you live. Organisations like Hidayah and Keshet exist for Muslim and Jewish LGBTQIA+ people too.

Books to help your child with sexuality anxiety		
Children	**Teens**	**Adults**
Grandad's Camper by Harry Woodgate The Girl with Two Dads by Mel Elliott And Tango Makes Three by Justin Richardson and Peter Parnell	Pride Power: The Young Person's Guide to LGBTQ+ Book by Harriet Dyer Queerly Autistic: The Ultimate Guide for LGBTQIA+ Teens on the Spectrum by Erin Ekins	The Queer Parent: Everything You Need to Know From Gay to Ze by Lotte Jeffs and Stuart Oakley Parenting Your LGBTQ+ Teen: A Guide to Supporting, Empowering, and Connecting with Your Child by Allan Sadac

We Are Family by Patricia Hegarty	*Queer: The Ultimate LQBTQ Guide for Teens* by Kathy Belge and Marke Bieschke	*Out: A Parent's Guide to Supporting Your LGBTQIA+ Kid Through Coming Out and Beyond* by John Sovec
What Does LGBT+ Mean?: A Guide for Young People (and Grown-Ups) by Olly Pike	*She Gets the Girl* by Rachael Lippincott and Alyson Derrick	*Uncommon Love: God's Heart for Christian Parents of Gay Kids* by Mary Comm
The Pirate Mums by Jodie Lancet-Grant		
'Twas the Night Before Pride by Joanna McClintick		*How to Stop Homophobic and Biphobic Bullying: A Practical Whole-School Approach* by Jonathan Charlesworth
From Archie to Zack by Vincent X. Kirsch		

Seventeen

Help! My Child's Panic Attacks Are Giving Me Anxiety!

Panic attacks are frightening for both children and parents. Above all, as parents, we want to protect our children from pain and fear – yet when your child is gripped by a panic attack, it seems as if they are experiencing both.

This chapter will give you the information you need to help you manage panic attacks and give you a plan to help put appropriate support in place until they stop completely.

What are panic attacks?

Panic attacks are a sudden-onset panic brought on by an episode of severe anxiety. The cause may be immediately obvious. Your child might be upset at having to separate from you or they have been confronted by something they fear: a big dog, a loud noise. However, panic attacks can also erupt for unfathomable reasons. You simply can't work out what has caused your child to suffer in this way. An inexplicable panic attack worries parents because they are not sure how to prevent it happening again.

Panic attacks come with physical symptoms that can be distressing to witness. These symptoms include:

- Feeling faint, dizzy or light-headed.
- Feeling nauseous.
- Abdominal discomfort.
- Chest pains and shortness of breath.
- Heart palpitations.
- Fluctuating body temperature.
- Hyperventilating.

The physical nature of panic attacks, which makes children (and often their parents) think there may be something medically wrong, adds to your child's fear they are in danger.

IMPORTANT: If your child has had any of these symptoms and you think it might be a panic attack, please visit your GP to confirm this and check that they are not suffering from any other medical condition.

How common are panic attacks and why do they happen?

Panic attacks are not common in young children. Frequency increases during adolescence.

Around 3–5 per cent of adolescents suffer from panic attacks and they are more common for girls than boys.

Panic attacks can happen because:

- Your child is stressed or overwhelmed.
- Your child has experienced a significant change recently.
- Your child has experienced loss.
- Your child is genetically predisposed to them as others in your family have had them.
- Your child is scared enough to bring on a flight or freeze response.
- Your child has been confronted by something that is their phobia or a fear.

What should I do in the moment when my child is having a panic attack?

When a child is having a panic attack, your job is to help your child know they will be OK and you will help them to calm down and deal with the situation.

Start by staying as calm as you can. Your child is going through something frightening and you want to fix it. You may also feel tense or embarrassed about other people seeing what's happening or trying to get involved.

Speak in a slow and calm voice. Make soft eye contact with your child. Imagine you know exactly what to do and try to project a sense of quiet confidence.

Try not to shout or show your frustration because your child is already highly stressed. Raising your voice will only make it more difficult for both of you to bring the attack to a close.

Tell your child you can see how hard and worrying this is but that you are here and you will be with them until they feel better.

> **Firework idea**
>
> **There is not a single case worldwide where a person has died from a panic attack. While scary for adults and children, there are no long-term medical dangers from having a panic attack. Knowing this fact can help both of you remain calm as you know that soon this will be over.**

When your child is having a panic attack, they are in survival mode. Your task is to show them that whatever the original reason for their distress, they are now safe and they can begin to slow down their breathing, stop crying or panting and return to their normal behaviour. You can do that by trying to engage their thinking brain – the prefrontal cortex – to help them manage the situation more practically and less emotionally. All the interventions below help a person in survival mode find safety or peace of mind. Talk them through with your child on a non-panicky day and then use them when they are in the thick of a panic attack.

Grounding techniques

A grounding technique is any action that draws the person's mind back to the present. It stops the brain catastrophising and focuses on what is going on right here, right now. Grounding techniques can be used to calm a panic attack or to stop one brewing in the first place.

Tried and trusted grounding techniques include:

Five Senses Check-in

Look for five things you can see, four things you can hear, three things you can touch, two things you can smell and one thing you can taste. (For examples, see page 177.)

Think Throughs

Ask a question that requires some thought, for example:

- If you had a private plane, where would you go?
- If you had £10 million, what would you buy?
- If you could have dinner with three famous people, who would you choose?
- If you had a shop, what would you sell?
- If you could have any animal as a pet, what would you choose?

These questions bring us back to the top part of our brain helping us separate from the panic in the present.

Slow Breathing

Slow breathing is helpful as it shows our body we are safe and we have time to be still and breathe. The opposite happens when we are scared, as we move flightily and become out of breath. Try these techniques:

- Box breathing – see page 175 for more information.
- Breathe in for five counts, hold for five then breathe out for six.
- Use a calming app.
- Watch a breathing video.

Physical Contact

Increasing physical contact can induce oxytocin and serotonin, which can directly counter the impact of the cortisol and adrenaline people produce during panic attacks. Create a feeling of safety with the following techniques:

- Use EFT tapping – this is a calming practice that can be learned quickly. It involves tapping specific points on the head, face, hands and chest. It's similar to meditation but you don't have to sit still and it also uses speech or affirmations to help calm the body.

- Use butterfly hug/taps – cross your arms and put your hands on your chest near the opposite shoulder; you can interlock your hands to make it look more like a butterfly. Then breathe deeply in and out. Then alternate patting each hand one at a time in a steady rhythm. You can do it harder or softer while breathing slowly in and out.
- Wrap your child in a blanket or a jumper.
- Use a fidget toy.
- Practise muscle tensing and relaxing.
- Use a comfort object.

Meet Their Needs

- Offer time away from you if they would rather be alone, but check on them and what they need.
- Help them drink water.
- Move your child to a safer location if necessary.

Distraction

- Use affirmations or calming phrases. Affirmations can be sentences to make you feel calm or empowered like 'I can manage anything', 'I am brave', or 'In a few minutes this will be over.' Or you might encourage them to say out loud a list of things, like the colours of the rainbow, album titles in order from their favourite artist or ingredients for a recipe they love. Anything that feels rhythmic or comforting.

- Listen to music.
- Sing or hum together.
- Watch a video that will distract your child.
- Let them be quiet while you tell them a funny story from your childhood.
- Go through the alphabet starting at A and encourage them to think of animals, fruit, countries, films that start with each letter.
- Count slowly to fifty.
- Help them visualise a safe or happy place or imagine the things that would make this situation better or feel safer.

What support is available for children who have panic attacks?

If your child is having regular panic attacks, it could indicate they are more severely affected by something than you realised and they need extra support. If they have been through something traumatic or life-changing without professional support, it may be time now to secure additional help.

- Consider therapy, counselling, CBT, EMDR or hypnotherapy for your child.
- Use this book to explore other possible causes for your child's anxiety.
- Visit your GP and ask for recommendations.
- Help your child manage their mental health with a schedule that helps them feel their best with enough sleep, food,

downtime, time in nature and exercise (see page 345 for an example of a self-care checklist).

- If their panic attacks are so severe and frequent their lives are being badly affected, it is time to ask your GP for a psychiatrist referral where they will evaluate the merits of taking medication to help manage the extreme emotions and fear behind the panic attack. They may offer SSRIs (selective serotonin reuptake inhibitors), benzodiazepines or beta blockers, depending on age, medical history and need. You could look these up before you go to understand a little more of what the doctor may say.
- Read books and learn about panic attacks and what's going on behind them.
- Let your school know your child has been struggling so they can support them during school hours.

Books to help your child with panic attacks		
Children	Teens	Adults
Pilar's Worries by Victoria M. Sanchez Too Much!: An Overwhelming Day by Jolene Gutiérrez	The Panic Workbook for Teens: Breaking the Cycle of Fear, Worry, and Panic Attacks by Debra Kissen, Bari Goldman Cohen and Kathi Fine Abitbol Your Survival Guide to Panic Attacks by Bev Aisbett	My Anxious Mind: A Teen's Guide to Managing Anxiety and Panic by Michael A. Tompkins and Katherine A. Martinez

Eighteen

My Child is Self-Harming and It's Giving Me Anxiety!

Self-harm – or deliberate self-harm (DSH) as it can be called in medical contexts – is a coping strategy some young people use to turn their emotional pain into a physical pain. Although it can be very difficult for others to understand, self-harming works by distracting them from their distressed emotional state or temporarily distracting them from what they are going through.

Self-harm can include skin picking, hair or eyelash plucking, scratching, cutting or burning the skin.

Why do children self-harm?

To Relieve Emotional Pain

When children self-harm, the body will make a small number of opioids, the body's own painkiller. When a child feels that they are in emotional pain, they can work out that cutting or hurting themselves provides a temporary sense of relief. Anxious children pick, pull and cut to make use of this unusual and unexpected protective mechanism. Self-harming alleviates the feeling of panic rising inside them for a short time.

Children may not understand the correlation, but they will notice the sense of relief so that when their anxiety escalates to what feels like an unbearable level on another day, they will begin to use self-harm as a coping strategy.

Anxious children realise self-harming steadies and calms their anxiety about being out of control or under threat. The sensation that an ominous threat is hanging over them is dramatic and terrifying. Experts compare it with the fear an animal experiences when it is about to be eaten by a predator.

Self-harm temporarily enables children to feel more like the predator than their prey. Instead of feeling powerless, picking, plucking, scratching, cutting or burning themselves delivers a sense of being in charge.

To the children inflicting it on themselves, self-harm seems an efficient way of soothing their anxiety. Of course, the adults who love and care for them can see that the danger clearly outweighs the benefit. In worst-case scenarios, self-harming can lead to worrying mistakes and permanent damage.

Firework idea

For children who are self-harming by skin picking – i.e. pulling broken skin off, causing bleeding – my first suggestion would be to ask your GP for a dermatology appointment. This will help heal the skin, leading to

less picking as there are no pieces of skin to pull. As the skin begins to calm down, your child should too, helping you support their mental health.

Self-Punishment

Some young people find themselves in situations where they feel as if everything in their lives has gone wrong. These children become depressed and start to believe that they themselves are the cause of their problems. This can lead to extreme self-loathing. To a child who feels they are responsible for all the unhappiness in their life, it can seem logical to 'punish' themselves by self-harming. This distressing reaction is often observed in children who have experienced abuse, bullying or an acute mental health crisis leading to social isolation.

A Cry for Help

Sometimes children who are struggling with emotional issues will want to signal, in a way which cannot be ignored, how extremely unhappy they are. They use self-harm because they know, once you discover what they are doing, you will definitely take steps to support them. In these children, self-harm is performative – they do it because they need to be seen hurting themselves. It's a clear route to showing you they are in pain.

Social Pressure

Young people may search for self-harming content, websites or groups on social media as a way to connect with other children and feel accepted. Sometimes the music they listen to or fashion they follow will be favoured by other children who self-harm. There is no direct pressure to self-harm, but distressed young people might pick up on trends or ideas which they feel encourages them to try it.

Social media companies have responded to pressure to make it harder to share and seek content about self-harm. For example, if you search 'self-harm' on TikTok a message comes up saying: 'You're not alone – if you or someone you know is having a hard time, help is always available.' Links to helpful resources and the Samaritans' number appear on your screen.

That said, an investigation conducted by an Irish newspaper found it took fourteen minutes for TikTok to present self-harm-related content to a fake account described as belonging to a thirteen-year-old. It is essential to set up parental controls on your child's devices. Seek help if you don't know how. Discuss your child's online life with them, and check out 141 for online courses for parents on internet safety. Look at the sites they are following. Explain that you are not being nosey or controlling. It's your job as a parent to protect and supervise your child in real life and online. Talk about the hazards and dangers springing up on social media. Chat about pressure that can be put on children to self-harm.

Fighting Numbness

Some children who are depressed will find that their low chemical levels feel like they are numb all the time. They have lost the positive sensations of life, which can lead to reckless behaviour and larger attempts to create chemical boosts. Self-harm can give a huge rush of chemicals like adrenaline and opioids which can help depressed and anxious people feel less numb for a short time.

> **Firework idea**
>
> **Fidget toys can be very helpful to keep picking hands busy – this year I heard about a new kind of fidget toy that can help with skin picking. It is called a 'Picky Pad' and it is silicone with beads inside that you can pick out and get the feeling of satisfaction and dopamine without pulling your own skin. For less than £5 it's worth a go!**

How common is it?

About one in five adolescents (20 per cent) in the UK have reported self-harming at some point in their lives.

For slightly younger children, the numbers are lower but still significant, with estimates suggesting that around 7 per cent of children aged eleven to sixteen have self-harmed.

Self-harm is more prevalent among girls than boys. Approximately 25 per cent of teenage girls have self-harmed, compared to around 10 per cent of teenage boys.

In positive news, around 90 per cent of self-harming children stop completely by adulthood.

What is the difference between self-harm and suicidality?

It's widely accepted by the World Health Organization, the International Society for the Study of Self Injury and other sources that around 70–90 per cent of self-harming children use self-harm as a coping strategy, not as a means to kill themselves.

It's important to note that we cannot know if our child is part of the other 10–30 per cent of young people harming with intent to take their own life. To this end, we have to be vigilant and keep this possibility in mind and make appropriate provision if needed.

What are the warning signs for self-harm?

- Alcohol and drug misuse.
- Previous mental health issues.
- Increased social isolation.
- Deterioration in self-care.
- Sudden poor school performance.

- Friendship or romantic struggles.
- Clear mood changes.
- Increased anger.
- Noticeable melancholy.
- Engaging in a social culture of self-harm.

What to do if your child is self-harming

Reach Out

Even limited interactions to show you have noticed something is not right – like, 'I can see you have been having a tough time lately, what's up?' – can help a child feel that you are on their team.

Create a Team Around Your Child

Adding more concerned adults who have different skill sets and relationships to the child will make a huge difference. Ask a close family friend, aunt or uncle, teacher, counsellor or therapist to reach out. This gives the child the feeling of containment and brings greater security to you as a parent that you will not miss anything.

Talk About Self-harm With Openness

When the time is right and your child has opened up to you or you notice something, be brave and speak without using euphemisms about the harm. Show your child you are not scared to talk about it and they do not have to feel ashamed.

Clear Your House of Dangerous Objects

If you think your child might be hurting themselves, go around your house and remove any object that could be used to harm. Drop them off at a friend's house or move them to a location where it would be hard to find them. Although self-harmers will aim to find a way if they have their sights set, those who haven't yet established a routine or a feeling of necessity may often be dissuaded by the difficulty of finding what they need.

Help Develop Healthy Coping Strategies

Once you have an open dialogue with your child about the self-harm, you can explain that although you understand why they are doing it, you cannot let them continue as the possibility for accident is too high. Look through the list of coping strategies below and try them out when your child is calmer first. Then if they seem useful, try them again when they are emotionally dysregulated to see which healthier methods could take the place of harm.

Address Underlying Issues

Children who are harming are doing it because they are in distress or have lost themselves somehow. To help support healthy progress, it is sensible to find therapeutic support for your child as soon as possible. Ask your school, GP or a charity for support to see what counselling or therapy may be available.

Educate Yourself and Your Child About Self-harm

Once you have understood the irregular physical feeling of benefit, calm and pain relief your child may feel after self-harm and the possible feelings behind it, you can educate them on the same information and more. Get information from your GP or charity websites to help them see that they can have the same sensation of release, relief or control from other, safer options.

Involve the School

It's always useful to let the school know when we have fears about our child's safety. This allows us to have more eyes on them when they are out of the house and the reassurance that we are not the only person looking out for them. The school may suggest in-school counselling or do a school-wide education programme on the dangers of self-harm. They might provide a mentor or help them engage in the school community.

Monitoring and Follow-up

Make sure to keep maintaining connection with your child throughout their recovery. Keep lines of communication open and make sure they know they can always come to you and you will meet them with kindness and without judgement.

Additional coping strategies

Once your child has engaged in the process to get better, what other coping strategies can you offer?

As a parent, your aim is to keep life ticking along despite this shocking news, so try to keep your child in their regular routine: going to school, sleeping, eating and socialising. At the same time, focus on these next steps:

- Find some therapeutic support: CBT and DBT (see pages 41 and 297) are particularly recommended for self-harm.
- Visit your GP.
- Make time for your own self-care.
- Remind your child that doing exercise regularly and when you feel overwhelmed can help you produce a stream of endorphins which can improve mood and energy levels and reduce the need to self-harm.
- Practising mindfulness can help children learn to feel their urges, thoughts and feelings and then let them pass – find mindfulness apps, meditation videos or a mindfulness practitioner to help focus your child's mind.
- Join a support group or an online forum for those aiming to stop.

- Use my self-care checklist (see page 345) to help your child get back to their best mental health possible. Aim to get at least three ticks a week in five boxes, for a minimum of three weeks.

Tailor your suggestions depending on your child's reason for distress

If you know what the feeling is that lies behind your child's compulsion to self-harm, you can suggest the following ideas:

- **If the primary feeling is anger:** Squeeze a stress ball, put on a loud or angry song and sing or shout along, tear up paper, shake your body, dance, do exercise.
- **If the primary feeling is relieving numbness:** Eat something spicy, book something in your diary that is both fun and a little scary like a high ropes course, smell something with a strong smell, have a cold shower, hold an ice cube, listen to some good music, talk to a friend.
- **If the primary feeling is sadness or emotional overwhelm:** Go out into nature, connect with someone by telling them how you feel, get a massage or a facial, listen to music you love, eat something delicious, watch a funny film with a friend, have a big cry and don't try to stop yourself, wrap yourself up in a blanket like a burrito, find someone you feel safe with to give you a hug.

- **If the primary feeling is looking for control:** Tidy your room, do a clear-out, write a list of things you need to do and then tick them off, make your body tight and then release it, set yourself a simple exercise goal and then try to meet it like walking for ten minutes a day, help in your house or garden.

- **If the primary feeling is shame:** Start a gratitude journal, work on mindful acceptance of your feelings, take a break from any friends, family or social media that make you feel bad about yourself, remind yourself you are not bad, you have had a hard time, spend time doing the things you are good at and see if you can be kind to yourself about your skill.

- **If the primary feeling is self-hatred and wanting to punish yourself:** Try to get moving, go to the gym, aim to remember things you used to love and do them, spend time with people who like you, use your feelings to create art and music.

Firework idea

Try not to swap one kind of self-harm for another even if it causes less damage. Some websites will suggest snapping a rubber band on your wrist instead of cutting, for example. But be aware it can actually become very addictive and can also damage skin and tendons in the wrist.

What should parents do in a crisis/emergency situation?

- Be ready to call the emergency services or take them to A&E immediately.
- Make sure to keep your GP in the loop.
- Aim to get your child therapeutic support as soon as possible.
- Look up the crisis intervention team number for your local area.
- Look into charities that support self-harmers and those with suicidal ideation.
- Where appropriate, inform other significant adults of this crisis and the plan to manage it.

Firework idea

In cases like this, it is better to be safe than sorry. Do not wait to get support, as soon as you feel fearful there may be a crisis on the way.

What support is available for children who self-harm?

- Mind provides information and support for anyone experiencing mental health issues, including self-harm.
- The National Self-Harm Network (NSHN) offers resources and support for individuals who self-harm.

- YoungMinds focuses on mental health support for young people and provides resources.
- Samaritans is a confidential helpline available 24/7 for anyone in emotional distress. You can reach them at 116 123.
- Self-Injury Support run a listening service you can call to talk about self-harm. They have great resources and an informative Instagram account @self_injury_support.
- Childline: for young people under nineteen, Childline offers support through various channels, including a helpline (0800 1111) and online chat.
- SHOUT is a text-based support service available 24/7 for anyone in crisis. You can text 'SHOUT' to 85258.
- Papyrus provides support for those self-harming and with suicidal ideation.

Books to help your child with self-harm
Stopping The Pain: A Workbook for Teens Who Cut and Self-Injure by Lawrence E. Shapiro
The DBT Skills Workbook for Teen Self-Harm: Practical Tools to Help You Manage Emotions and Overcome Self-Harming Behaviors by Sheri van Dijk
When Teens Self-Harm: How Parents, Teachers and Professionals Can Provide Calm and Compassionate Support by Monika Parkinson, Kerstin Thirlwall and Lucy Willetts
Can I Tell You About Self-Harm?: A Guide for Friends, Family and Professionals by Pooky Knightsmith

Conclusion

Help! I've Solved All My Problems. How Do I Calm Down Enough to Enjoy It?

Anxiety can be addictive. Everyone tells us parenthood is a minefield in which we lurch from crisis to crisis. We become used to being in a perpetual state of panic. One minute we're coping with chickenpox. The next we've lost our child's book bag and we're so exhausted from endless nights of broken sleep we can't remember where we put it. We are fraught and run ragged, living on our last nerve. In fact, we are so stressed we completely forget to notice when the day dawns and everything is calm. No one has a runny nose. Everyone slept through the night. All the children are happy at school and there's nothing at all to worry about.

So, I am reminding you in this final chapter of my book that sometimes anxiety ebbs away and it's a good policy to notice when that happens. Stop and take stock. You're not averting an emergency. Everything is running smoothly. This is the time to breathe deeply, congratulate yourself on a great job and take a moment to think about what you most enjoy in life and how to incorporate some of it into your routine.

Some positive ideas to help you find calm

Make Space for Yourself in Your Schedule

You can start small with a cup of delicious fragrant coffee on a bench in the sun, an unputdownable novel or a catch-up with a positive, fun friend. Or you can start big with a trip you have been hoping to take with your partner or a friend or investing in yourself by doing a course or learning a new skill. The sky's the limit.

Cut Down on Your To-do List

Here's how: try using the ABCDE method. Make your normal to-do list as usual then use the ABCDE method to label the things on your list.

- A – Must-dos. These are critical tasks that have serious consequences if not completed.
- B – Should-dos. These tasks are important but have minor consequences if delayed.
- C – Nice-to-dos. Tasks in this category have no significant consequences if left undone.
- D – Delegate.
- E – Eliminate.

For example, your list might look like this:

- Go to the dentist – B.
- Pick up dry cleaning – D.

- Get new uniform for Simon – A.
- Rewrite the presentation for Monday's meeting – A.
- Order new tiles for downstairs loo – B.
- Pick up milk – D.
- Order a birthday present for Lucy – C.
- Organise family dinner for reading week – C.
- Look up tickets to see Coldplay – C.
- Organise coffee with Phoebe – C.
- Get new wellies if it's meant to rain this weekend – E.

This system immediately shows us what is important for work and family, but also what we are excited to do in our lives and what to make time for. It's a fast way to set priorities and maintain the most enjoyable parts of our lives.

Reclaim Your Identity

Who are you? Who were you? Who do you want to be now? What matters to you? Where do you feel the most like your-self? What do you miss about your younger self?

Work up the courage to be brave and believe you are entitled and able to start new things, go out for the fun of it and revisit things you used to love, to help find out who you are now. This is your life and you – even if you are a mum/dad/son/daughter/worker or partner – are allowed to be the star.

Start Rituals and Traditions and Book Time for Love

The families I work with often say they never spend enough time just having fun with their children – particularly their teenagers.

If that's your situation, why not think about rituals and traditions? Any family can make up its own ones. They have nothing to do with religion and everything to do with making special unified moments the whole family can enjoy together on a regular basis. Rituals need rules, tools and significance.

For example: measure your children's height on the same doorpost the night before they start the new school year. Make a ceremony out of it. Have something delicious to eat afterwards. Make sure your family measuring ceremony is done in exactly the same way each time. Use a special ceremonial pen. Mark each child's growth in their favourite colour. Take a picture of the family on Measuring Day. Everyone must be there. This is a milestone your family takes seriously. You look forward to it. You count down the days till Measuring Day. It has significance because it marks the passing of time. It is a particular tradition unique to your family. It is something everyone participates in together.

Here are a few more ideas to get you started:

- Once a year, give your child a vote on a family trip.

- Host weekly/monthly game nights. Keep score in a special notebook. Have small prizes for the winners. Foster an atmosphere of fun and competition.
- Plan weekly/monthly movie nights. Everyone in the family has a turn to choose their favourite. Bring in squashy cushions and popcorn and make sure the curtains are closed for a cinematic atmosphere.
- Interview your child the night before their birthday each year.
- Host a back-to-school/Halloween/Easter egg hunt/party.
- Make a folder for your child and add drawings and schoolwork to it. At the end of the year, get out the Blu Tack and set up a gallery of their best work. Walk round the exhibition viewing their work and discuss how much you are enjoying it.
- Write your child a secret letter at the end of every school year and give them to them when they leave school or college.
- Plan to go away on one special trip with your child before they are eighteen.
- Have a family celebration day – commemorate a great family event every year.
- Art day – once a year take your kids to do something creative.
- Family Olympics – invite your extended family over for an Olympic-style sports day!
- Monthly 'kids cook dinner'.
- Invent a secret family handshake. Don't tell anyone.

- Say goodnight and good morning in a special way.
- Challenge your child to read as many books as possible, stack them up (or measure how big each one is and add them up) and when the tower is taller than your child, buy them a present – another book!
- Hold a monthly family meeting to discuss likes, dislikes, gripes, rules and plans. Even the youngest has an equal say.
- Host a monthly 'bring a friend' picnic.
- Enjoy special time where one parent takes just one child to enjoy something simple but fun.
- Celebrate the seasons with seasonal hunts.
- New year's resolutions or letters.

Then try to remember to do them and make memories while putting real smiles on everyone's faces!

Be Brave Enough to Ask for Help

Ask for help if you need it. Everyone needs support. You cannot juggle everything alone. At home or at work, pluck up the courage to ask for whatever you need to make life easier. No one will think any less of you. In fact, people will respect you for making your needs clear and enlisting help to achieve your goals.

Be Confident About How Great You Are!

You are the only you. No one will ever be anything like you. That is an enormous deal. You are an enormous deal. There are skills, ideas, memories, personality traits and plans inside you that will never be released into the world if you don't let them out.

Think of it this way: 'If you don't say how great you are, who will?!'

At work, it's impossible for our bosses to know all we have accomplished and praise us or promote us if we don't tell them.

Our partners can't sing our praises if they don't notice what we've achieved. We have to tell them.

We cannot inspire our children to be as awesome as we are if we don't tell them our life story and emphasise our achievements. If you want to be your children's inspiration, you must do something inspirational and make sure you tell your children all about it! Just occasionally, blow your own trumpet as hard as you can.

Make More Positive Chemicals

If your life feels grey and monotonous, help your brain make more positive chemicals by doing the following:

- Prioritising good sleep.
- Getting out of the house into the light for at least thirty minutes a day – preferably in a green space.
- Eating enough good food to fuel your body and varying your diet to improve your gut health.

- Making time to do things you love.
- Moving your body.
- Seeing people who make you smile.
- Drinking enough water.
- Giving your body time to sit and relax.
- Trying to have some physical fun (sex is definitely recommended if possible!).

All these measures help create the chemicals we need to stay happy, healthy and connected.

Be Kind and Compassionate to Yourself

We all have capacity to be our own worst critic. Whether you grew up with critical parents, feel like the least capable person in your family or didn't meet your own expectations, you will have an internal voice that often makes you feel inadequate.

Now is the time to reclaim your inner voice and change it from critic to hype man!

It's easy to do. Back yourself. Be your own team leader. Don't say, 'Why would they pick me?' You are just as capable as the other candidates. Don't accuse yourself of sitting on your bum and being lazy. You have been rushing around all day and just need to relax.

The more you silence that vicious inner voice, the more the kinder, fairer one will be heard. Soon you will believe you have the capacity to fulfil your ambitions.

When Parenting, Think, 'If I Were in This Situation, What Do I Wish Someone Would Do for Me?'

As parents we cannot get everything right and will never know whether we did or didn't do the right thing, but one thing we can do is act with kindness. When our child is upset, angry, lonely, embarrassed, heartbroken, confused or excited, think, 'If I were in that situation, what would I hope someone would do for me? I'm sure I would want empathy, acknowledgement and a bit of their time so that is something I can give to my child now.'

It's a good way to use your humanity and experience to support your child no matter what.

Suspend Disbelief, Find Magic and Fun

This book has been a pleasure to write. I've loved thinking about you and your child. I hope I've been able to ease your anxiety by helping you come up with constructive strategies. I hope you've become the loving security guard your child needs to fight off the spectre of fear that has been causing them distress.

I hope you imagine me smiling at my laptop when I think of children going back to school, grieving healthily, expressing their real selves without fear, feeling looked after and seen by their empathetic, loving parent. I breathe more deeply when I think of all the parents who might be able to relax and feel empowered as they see their child's anxiety melt away.

I also want you to know there is life and fun out there for your families and yourself. Don't forget to sing along to the radio, have a laugh playing games together, splash in puddles and spot the magic in the world. There is so much wonder to share with your child. You just have to remember to look out the window and find it.

Remember you are not alone.

As I always say, 'It's OK not to be OK, but you don't have to stay that way!'

Find the support you need to live the most beautiful life you can.

I wish you well, always.

Only Ever as Happy as Your Least Happy Child

If what they say is true and I will never again be happier than you are,

Then I will work to rebuild your smile when it crumbles, with stories and memories from our happiest days.

I will unburden your arms as you are weighed down, then watch my strength grow as it did when I carried you in my arms.

Help! My Child's Anxiety is Giving Me Anxiety

I will paint pictures, sing songs, dance with you around the kitchen and watch as you take the distracted path back to yourself.

I will raise the portcullis when I am sure no danger is near and teach you how to open doors and stand bravely in the face of foes.

I will model compassion and learn to see perfection in the magic mistakes we have made and the surprises that arrived in our lives because of them.

All your favourite things will forever be written on my heart even when you have long forgotten them.

I will remember those who said you couldn't play or called you nasty names even when the break-time bell has rung for the last time.

I will stand tall and protect you from avalanches and rainstorms and, if I can, I will take myself to safety too. We can sit in the thick dark, huddled in our love until the sun comes and we can regain our strength.

If, as they say, my smile, my world, my life will never be bigger than you . . . I will be proud all the days of my life that I had a part in the story of you and you rewrite the story of me.

And even though I know I will never be a perfect parent,

Saskia Joss

I will give my all to giving you all I can and hope you know that's what I did.

The love between us is always strong and the life between us stronger still.

It's a job I'm willing to take, it's an adventure I'd pay for, it's the dream I wished I would live and now I do.

With love,
From me x

Acknowledgements

Writing a book was not on my bucket list. I didn't even dare to dream of being an author. I was so sure it would never happen. I'm a late diagnosed dyslexic, brimming with ideas. I can vividly express my thoughts verbally, but find it much more difficult to write them down. It seemed impossible that I, who battled to commit my insights to paper, would ever succeed in creating a book designed to help struggling parents. I'd like to thank everyone who allowed me to believe I had something important enough to say and was more than capable of expressing myself in paragraphs. Producing this book truly has made my dreamiest dreams come true!

I'd like to thank Anna Steadman for her clairvoyance and vision. Anna, you saw me lecturing and spotted a quality in me which convinced you I had the capacity to reach out to a wider audience. Thank you for your unwavering confidence and enthusiasm, coupled with your ability to spur me on and guide me through the process. I have loved working with you. It has been a calm and hopeful pleasure.

Thank you to my mother, Vanessa. In raising me, you showed me how to create the safe environment this book helps families build. You helped me shape this book, came up with the title and used your experience of parenting and literary talent to make this the book I imagined. I love you and am so thankful for our life of adventures including this one. Here's to all the universe brings us.

Marc, you believed I could write a book when I was sure I couldn't. You were my steadfast supporter when training to be a therapist seemed like a crazy pipe dream. You make me feel as if I can accomplish anything and make the practical arrangements to make my ambitions viable. You are so kind, clever and funny. You provide love, perfect puns and facilitate the adventures which are now part of the beautiful story of our life together. I couldn't do what I do without you and I wouldn't want to. You are my favourite friend and my forever love.

Thank you to Lindsay Davies: as I was told you would, you took my book and made it clear, neat and more human and then tied it up with a gorgeous bow with your generous comments and humour. I was lucky indeed to have my book end up in your lap; what a win!

My wonderful Amiel and my spectacular Cecily: being your mummy has made my life magical, passionate and sparkly with promise. Reading, singing, dancing, creating every-thing with you is my favourite thing. Your kindness and excitement about the world infuse me with enthusiasm. Your kisses, cuddles, hair-stroking and tummy-squashing fill my heart and soul. I hope this book allows other parents to forget their worries and make time to enjoy their children as much as I enjoy and love you both unconditionally and with the zeal for life that you teach me. Know that I will always be here to be a security guard, ally, helper and cheerleader for you. As I always say, you could be forty-five and living in Australia – if you need me, I will be there.

My sister and best friend, Allegra, thank you for being my fiercest confidante, protector and inspiration. I have always wanted to be like you and being your sibling is the greatest luck. You are a light in the world and so are your marvellous children Zekey and Neroli. You are a remarkable mother. So many ideas here stem from watching you raise such smart, loving and golden people.

Thank you to my indomitable, funny, stylish and fabulous mother-in-law, Karen. You have taught me so much and brought laughter and *spinacha* too. Thank you for your babysitting skills, art classes and chess tutorials. Love you.

My incredible friends have been so kind. When I told my best friend Harriet there was an online listing for the book, before I could open the next message, she had already bought a pre-ordered copy. Laura told me she couldn't wait to brag about her author friend. Svetlana offered to proofread the whole thing before I had written a word. Fran, a highly regarded educator, said she would ask the schools she works in to invite me to give talks. My peppy friend Marian said she would organise a mum's meet-up so I could share my book. My friends helped me believe in myself. Their support means more than they know.

A special thank you to all the knowledgeable therapists who shared their expertise. Talya Ressel, Lubna Dar, Orla Muriel Blakelock and Jamie Crabb, you broadened my scope and expanded my insight. It was a pleasure working with you.

The biggest and most important thank you is for all the inspirational children I have worked with over the last fifteen years. It has been a privilege to sit next to you in your darkest days and stand aside with satisfaction as you no longer need me. Although I do not share real stories, my book is seasoned with information I learned from children and parents. I love my job because of the hard-working, loving families I work with. Thank you for trusting me with your whole world.

A final thank you to my wise mentors in education and therapy. I am so lucky to have learned from the best. Thank you to my unstoppable boss Christopher Flathers and all the outstanding teachers at the Orion and Goldbeaters schools. Thank you to Catherine Goodwin and Catherine Landucci for teaching me so much about the kind and caring way to educate children. Thank you to Alexandra Cooper whose passion for mental health brought me to St Michael's School to provide lectures for parents, where I met Anna (my editor) and so started the adventure of this book. Thank you to therapeutic wizards, Méabh Lynagh, Heather Gibson, Pretish Raja-Helm and all the empowering therapists at our dynamic practice, the Mill Hill Therapy Hub. I see you all work miracles every day. It is an honour to work with and learn from you all.

Follow me on Facebook, Instagram and TikTok @saskiajoss-therapy for more information about the book, parenting, mental health and neuroscience. Find out about the other work I do at www.saskiajosstherapy.co.uk

Glossary

Amygdala: A part of the brain that assesses danger and sets up your reaction in life-threatening situations.

Attachment Theory: The theory that explains how early relationships with parents and caregivers shape how we form bonds and trust others later in life.

BACP/UKCP/BAPT: Some of the professional bodies that therapists and counsellors in the UK must be registered with to practise.

- **BACP**: British Association for Counselling and Psychotherapy
- **UKCP**: UK Council for Psychotherapy
- **BAPT**: British Association of Play Therapists

Comorbidity: When a person has two or more health problems at the same time, such as anxiety and depression. It is often used to describe conditions that are more likely to present together.

Cortisol: The stress hormone your body releases when in danger or under pressure. It is needed to remind us of our limits, tell us what we are excited about, but it also makes us feel anxious. The overproduction of cortisol makes us feel anxious and gives us many of the physical symptoms that we see in anxious adults and children.

Dopamine: One of our positive-feeling brain chemicals, which incentivises us to work hard and gives us the feeling of a reward for successful tasks.

Dysregulated: When someone is overwhelmed by feelings, memories or sensory stimuli. They may need help to calm down or regain the feeling of control.

EBSA (Emotionally Based School Avoidance): School refusal triggered by anxiety or other emotional issues.

EHCP (Education, Health and Care Plan): A legal plan for a child's education decided by a school, a Sendco and the local council that should outline all the specialist provisions needed to support a child's emotional or educational needs. UK specific terminology. Only organised for children with more complex special needs.

Endorphins: A positive chemical made in the brain as an incentive and reward for moving/exercise.

Fight or Flight Response: The Fight or Flight response, sometimes including Freeze or Fawn, is an automatic response that our bodies make to threat to life. If a bear broke into the room, your brain would decide whether your best chance of survival was to fight it, run, hide or pretend to be dead. Once the threat has passed, we are meant to calm down. Anxiety is a lingering sensation that the threat has not really passed.

GAD (Generalised Anxiety Disorder): The diagnosis given to a person who is chronically anxious about everything in their life and cannot find comfort.

Highly Sensitive Child: A child who is more impacted by daily life. They notice sounds, smells, textures, changes in schedule more acutely and seem to feel more deeply or have more extreme reactions. This may be due to their natural personality or because of neurodivergence or sensory processing issues.

IEP (Individual Education Plan): A personalised plan for a child in school who needs extra support with learning or behaviour, usually set up by the Sendco, the class teacher and the parent/carer.

Neurodiversity/Neurodivergent: A relatively new term to classify those with brains that work in a different way. It is a more inclusive and factual term for people with autism, ADHD, dyslexia, dyspraxia and other similar educational learning difficulties.

Occupational Therapy (OT): A type of physical therapy that helps people improve core skills like balance, self-care, processing and understanding. It is the logistical support that many children need to progress through developmental milestones and become more independent.

Oxytocin: A hormone sometimes called the 'love hormone', we make it when we feel a connection between us and another person. It is the only reciprocal chemical our body makes, which means if you are feeling liked and loved by someone, they could be too. It is the chemical that bonds babies and caregivers and keeps us getting up in the middle of the night to care and connect with them.

Polyvagal Theory: A theory by Stephen Porgess that explains that we get our sense of safety and connection from information sent from all over our body, from our face to our gut. The polyvagal nerve gives us data that tells us if we can 'rest and digest' – relax and continue our day or we need to 'Fight or flight' to save ourselves from danger. This idea underpins what we know about anxiety.

Proprioception: Your body's ability to sense where it is in space. Are you close to the wall, or will you bang into something if you move? Interestingly, we have learnt that better proprioceptive sense helps children relax and decreases hypervigilance.

SENDCo/SENCo: The professional in a UK school who helps students with special educational needs and disabilities (SEND).

Serotonin: A brain chemical that regulates mood. It brings us back to a more even mood after big feelings, whether positive or negative.

Window of Tolerance: The theory by Dan Siegal sets out that we all have a level of things we can manage without getting overwhelmed. This changes regularly, based on other factors in our environment like tiredness, stress or injury.

References

Abraham, E., & Feldman, R. (2014), 'The Neural Basis of Parental Caregiving: Implications for Parent–Child Bonding and Emotional Regulation', *Journal of Child Psychology and Psychiatry* 55(4), 407–17

Ainsworth, M. D. S., Blehar, M.C., Waters, E. & Wall, S. (1978), *Patterns of Attachment: A Psychological Study of the Strange Situation*, Lawrence Erlbaum Associates

Algoe, S. B., Haidt, J., & Gable, S. L. (2008), 'Beyond Reciprocity: Gratitude and Relationships in Everyday Life', *Emotion* 8(3), 425–9

Biddulph, S. (2010), *The New Manhood: The Handbook for a New Kind of Man*, Finch Publishing

Boyce, T. (2019), *The Orchid and the Dandelion: Why Some Children Struggle and How All Can Thrive*, Random House

Breedlove, S. M., Watson N. V., & Rosenzweig, M. (2013), *Biological Psychology: An Introduction to Behavioral, Cognitive, and Clinical Neuroscience*, Sinauer Associates, Inc

Bushak, L. (2022), 'Nearly 84% of Mental Health Videos on TikTok are Misleading: Study', *Medical Marketing and Media*, available at: www.mmm-online.com/home/channel/nearly-84-of-mental-health-videos-on-tiktok-are-misleading-study/ [accessed 29 September 2024]

Campbell, D. (12 March 2024), 'Children to stop getting puberty blockers at gender identity clinics, says NHS England', *Guardian*

Carr, P. B., & Walton, G. M. (2014), 'Cues of Working Together Fuel Intrinsic Motivation', *Journal of Experimental Social Psychology* 53, 169–84. DOI: 10.1016/j.jesp.2014.03.015

Chang, A. M., Aeschbach, D., Duffy, J. F., & Czeisler, C. A. (2015), 'Evening Use of Light-emitting eReaders Negatively Affects Sleep, Circadian Timing, and Next-morning Alertness', *Proceedings of the National Academy of Sciences* 112(4), 1232–7. DOI: 10.1073/pnas.1418490112

Davison, K. K., et al. (2011), 'Activity-related Support from Parents, Peers, and Siblings and Adolescents' Physical Activity: Are There Gender Differences?', *Journal of Physical Activity and Health* 8.6: 791–9

Davison, K. K., et al. (2016), 'Fathers' Representation in Observational Studies on Parenting and Childhood Obesity:

A Systematic Review and Content Analysis', *International Journal of Behavioral Nutrition and Physical Activity* 13.1: 1–13

Epel, E. S., Blackburn, E. H., Lin, J., Dhabhar, F. S., Adler, N. E., Morrow, J. D., & Cawthon, R. M. (2004), 'Accelerated Telomere Shortening in Response to Life Stress', *Proceedings of the National Academy of Sciences* 101(49), 17312–15

Harris, T. A. (1969), *I'm OK – You're OK*, Harper & Row

Higuchi, S., Motohashi, Y., Liu, Y., & Maeda, A. (2005), 'Effects of VDT Tasks with a Bright Display at Night on Melatonin, Core Temperature, and Sleepiness', *Journal of Applied Physiology* 98(1), 177–84. DOI: 10.1152/japplphysiol.00172.2004

Hoekzema, E., et al. (2017), 'Parenting: Brain Structure and Function in Human Mothers and Fathers', *Neuropsychologia* 105, 65–79

Jacobs, T. L., et al. (2011), 'Intensive Meditation Training, Immune Cell Telomerase Activity, and Psychological Mediators', *Psychoneuroendocrinology* 36(5), 664–81

Jenni, O. G., Fuhrer, H. Z., Iglowstein, I., Molinari, L., & Largo, R. H. (2005), 'A Longitudinal Study of Bed Sharing and Sleep Problems Among Swiss Children in the First 10 Years of Life', *Pediatrics* 115(1), 233–40

Kim, P., Leckman, J. F., Mayes, L. C., Feldman, R., Wang, X., & Swain, J. E. (2010), 'The Plasticity of Human Maternal

Brain: Longitudinal Changes in Brain Anatomy During the Early Postpartum Period', *Behavioral Neuroscience* 124(5), 695–700

Lally, P., van Jaarsveld, C. H. M., Potts, H. W. W., & Wardle, J. (2010), 'How Are Habits Formed: Modelling Habit Formation in the Real World', *European Journal of Social Psychology* 40(6), 998–1009. DOI: 10.1002/ejsp.674

Lazarus, J. (2021), 'Negativity Bias: An Evolutionary Hypothesis and an Empirical Programme', *Learning and Motivation* 75, 101731. DOI: 10.1016/j.lmot.2021.101731

Mercer, J. (2014), 'Infant Routines and the Role of Predictability in Development', *Journal of Infant Behavior and Development* 37(1), 1–10

Miller, L. J., Anzalone, M. E., Lane, S. J., Cermak, S. A., & Osten, E. T. (2007), 'Concept Evolution in Sensory Integration: A Proposed Nosology for Diagnosis', *American Journal of Occupational Therapy* 61(2), 135–40. DOI: 10.5014/ajot.61.2.135

Mindell, J. A., Leichman, E. S., DuMond, C., & Sadeh, A. (2017), 'Sleep and Social-emotional Development in Infants and Toddlers', *Journal of Clinical Child & Adolescent Psychology* 46(2), 236–46

Morgan, C., et al. (2017), 'Incidence, Clinical Management, and Mortality Risk following Self Harm among Children and Adolescents: Cohort Study in Primary Care', *British Medical Journal* 359

National Center for Transgender Equality (2015), *The Report of the 2015 U.S. Transgender Survey*, retrieved from ncte.org

Newman, S. (2022), 'Best Age for Kids to Start Doing Chores', *Psychology Today*, available at: www.psychologytoday.com/gb/blog/singletons/202211/best-age-for-kids-to-start-doing-chores [accessed 27 September 2024]

NHS Digital (2018), *Mental Health of Children and Young People in England, 2017: Summary of Key Findings*, available at: https://digital.nhs.uk/data-and-information/publications/statistical/mental-health-of-children-and-young-people-in-england/2017/2017 [accessed 10 August 2024]

NICABM (n.d.), 'How to Help Your Clients Understand Their Window of Tolerance', available at: www.nicabm.com/trauma-how-to-help-your-clients-understand-their-window-of-tolerance/ [accessed 27 September 2024]

O'Connor, M.-F., Wellisch, D. K., Stanton, A. L., Eisenberger, N. I., Irwin, M. R., & Lieberman, M. D. (2008), 'Craving Love? Complicated Grief Activates Brain's Reward Center', *Neuroimage* 42(2), 969–72. DOI: 10.1016/j.neuroimage.2008.04.256

Owens, J. A., Jones, C., & Nash, R. (2010), 'Sleep and Television Viewing in Children and Adolescents, *Sleep Medicine* 11(2), 187–91

Paul, I. M., Johnson, S. L., Goodman, W., & Qin, X. (2012), 'The Interventionist Co-sleeping Study', *Pediatrics* 130(3), 450–8

Puterman, E., Lin, J., Blackburn, E., O'Donovan, A., Adler, N., & Epel, E. (2010), 'The Power of Exercise: Buffering the Effect of Chronic Stress on Telomere Length', *PLoS One* 5(5), e10837

Queensland Brain Institute (2018), 'Hippocampus: Where are Memories Stored in the Brain?', University of Queensland, available at: https://qbi.uq.edu.au/brain-basics [accessed 13 May 2024]

Robertson, J. & Bowlby, J. (1952), 'Responses of Young Children to Separation from their Mothers', *Courrier du Centre International de l'Enfance* 2(13), 131–40

Robinson, L., & Segal, J. (2017), 'Mood-Boosting Power of Dogs', available at: https://hr.unm.edu/docs/ehp/mood-boosting-power-of-dogs.pdf [accessed 12 July 2024]

Scaglioni, S., et al. (2018), 'Factors Influencing Children's Eating Behaviours', *Nutrients* 10.6: 706

Schaaf, R. C., & Nightlinger, K. M. (2007), 'Occupational Therapy Using a Sensory Integrative Approach: A Case Study of Effectiveness', *American Journal of Occupational Therapy* 61(2), 239–46. DOI: 10.5014/ajot.61.2.239

Šimić, G., et al. (2021), 'Understanding Emotions: Origins and Roles of the Amygdala', *Biomolecules*, 11(6):823. DOI: 10.3390/biom11060823

Sipler, E. (2020), 'Making Our Nervous System Work for Us Using the Polyvagal Theory to Improve Our

Wellbeing', South Eastern Health and Social Care Trust, available at: https://setrust.hscni.net/wp-content/uploads/2023/02/Nervous-System-Brochure-Final.pdf [accessed 27 September 2024]

Spokas, M. & Heimberg, R. (2009), 'Overprotective Parenting, Social Anxiety, and External Locus of Control: Cross-sectional and Longitudinal Relationships', *Cognitive Therapy and Research* 33, 543–51. DOI: 10.1007/s10608-008-9227-5

Structural Learning (2023), 'Bowlby's Attachment Theory: Understanding the Importance of Early Emotional Bonds', available at: www.structural-learning.com [accessed 3 June 2024]

The Trevor Project (2021), *The Trevor Project National Survey on LGBTQ Youth Mental Health 2021*, available at thetrevorproject.org [accessed 25 August 2024]

Tompkins, C. (2021), 'A Spoonful, Not a Flood: Dosing 101', Arizona Association for Foster and Adoptive Parents, available at: www.azafap.org/uncategorized/a-spoonful-not-a-flood-dosing-101/ [accessed 9 May 2024]

Touchette, É., Petit, D., Séguin, J. R., Boivin, M., Tremblay, R. E., & Montplaisir, J. Y. (2007), 'Associations Between Sleep Duration Patterns and Behavioral/Cognitive Functioning at School Entry', *Sleep* 30(9), 1213–19

Trost, S. G., et al. (2007), 'Physical Activity in Children and Adolescents', *American Journal of Health Promotion* 21.4 (2007): 307–13

van der Bruggen, C. D. A., Bögels, S. M., & Muris, P. (2010), 'The Relationship Between Child and Parent Anxiety and Parental Control: A Meta-Analytic Review', *Journal of Child Psychology and Psychiatry* 51(4), 428–40

Xiong, Y., Hong, H., Liu, C., et al. (2023), 'Social Isolation and the Brain: Effects and Mechanisms', *Molecular Psychiatry* 28, 191–201. DOI: 10.1038/s41380-022-01835-w

Yeung, S. K., & Lau, E. Y. H. (2019), 'Overprotective Parenting and Child Anxiety: The Role of Cognitive Biases and Child Effortful Control', *Journal of Family Psychology* 33(3), 292–302

YoungMinds (2018), 'Addressing Adversity: Prioritising Childhood to Address Adversity', available at: https:// youngminds.org.uk/media/2186/youngminds-addressing-adversity.pdf [accessed 10 August 2024]

Index